PRA

D0498781

"This book is written from the .... to help its readers get to the depth of their Casa visit before they arrive. A Casa visit is so much more than adhering to the protocols. It is a chance to open hearts and minds to personal miracles. This book is a perfect tool for finding the inner connection and opening to an experience of the highest benefit possible. Thank you, Mytrae, for writing this book. It is, indeed, a true gift for the reader."

—Diana Rose
Casa Guide
www.miraclesofjohnofgod.com

"For the outer trip to John of God there are a number of good books to help the traveler. But the inner journey of healing is far more complex, subtle and mysterious. Only a trained psychotherapist and spiritual guide familiar with the depths of the inner world could write such a book. This is the best guide for the inner journey of healing at the Casa de Dom Inácio."

—Brant Cortright, Ph.D.
Author of *Psychotherapy and Spirit*
Psychologist and Professor at California Institute of Integral
Studies, San Francisco

"Based on her frequent trips to the Casa de Dom Inácio, Mytrae has a wonderful way of encompassing practical advice within a style of writing that effuses compassion and love for the reader. Ultimately, John of God's work involves healing of the heart and soul. Mytrae's heart and soul truly reach out to touch the reader in a manner that will only enhance the healing you receive at the Casa. I only wish that Mytrae's book was available a few years ago when I made my trip to Brazil to see John of God."

—Michael Quinn
Crystal Bed Owner

"I'm very pleased to see that Mytrae offers the best of a detail-oriented approach *and* a heart approach in this wonderful and thorough manual for people wanting to be well-prepared before visiting the Casa! This manual will not only help people avoid a lot of the confusion that first-time visitors often experience, but will also assist in helping them get more out of their time there than they may have been able to achieve otherwise. As helping people maximize their experience at the Casa is a goal I share with Mytrae, I fully endorse her work!!!"

—Josie RavenWing
Casa Guide and Author of
The Book of Miracles: The Healing Work of João de Deus
www.johnofgod-brazil.net

JOHN

A GUIDE TO YOUR HEALING JOURNEY

OF

WITH SPIRIT DOCTORS BEYOND THE VEIL

GOD

MYTRAE MELIANA

blue
leopard
press

san francisco

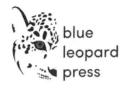
blue
leopard
press

Blue Leopard Press

John of God: A Guide to Your Healing Journey with Spirit Doctors Beyond the Veil
Mytrae Meliana

The information contained in this book is intended to be educational and not for diagnosis, prescription, or treatment of any health disorder whatsoever. This information should not replace consultation with a competent health professional. The content of this book is intended to be used as an adjunct to a rational and responsible healthcare program prescribed by a professional healthcare practitioner. The author is in no way liable for any misuse of the material.

Copyeditor: Kelly O'Connor McNees
Cover design: Kathleen Finch/Black Kat Design
Front cover photos: Karen Leffler Photography
Interior design: The Roberts Group

Published in the United States of America

ISBN 978-0-9914606-0-1

CONTENTS

CONTENTS

FOREWORD

A VISIT TO JOHN of God's Casa de Dom Inácio opens innumerable doors to growth and healing. It is truly a place of miracles. In my nine years as a Casa guide and in my life as an author, I spend a lot of time talking to people about healing. I have seen people come in with many questions and misunderstandings. With or without a guide, the best benefits come from preparation for the amazing journey on which one has embarked.

People ask me, "Who heals and how? What is happening when we don't heal? How do we best invite the healing that we seek?"

People come to the Casa seeking healing on physical, emotional, and spiritual levels, and can co-create that healing with the Entities. But traditional "healing" is a linear path. That's valuable, but as a teacher of non-duality and meditation, I also address the question in a different way. That which is aware of illness is not ill. That which is aware of anger is not angry; that which is aware of fear is not afraid. With our inner practice we find the balance of compassion for the suffering human that *is* afraid and in pain, no denial; and the ability to rest in and trust the ever-healed, the innate radiant perfection of our being.

I was delighted to receive an advance copy of *John of God*

from Mytrae Meliana and the request to write this foreword. We have been waiting for this book. The journey to John of God and to healing starts the minute we form the intention to travel there. The Entities begin to help us. Mytrae's words clarify the path.

Her explanations and guidance on the process of preparing for the journey are clear and loving, just what I want for my groups. She asks the reader to go deep, to find the inner conditions that have shaped our ailments, and to trust our ability to move on. This is courageous work that asks a lot of us but is the path to true healing. Her guidance walks the reader through with questions that help the heart to open. While the book is for the person about to journey to see John of God, it will also serve many people who are on a healing journey but unable to make that trip to Brazil.

Mytrae carefully points out that the Entities do half the work, but we must do the other half. Are we ready? What's holding us back? Are there habitual stories of unworthiness or distortion to which we hold? What resistance do we have to opening to the fullest possible healing, to expressing what we seek?

We co-create with spirit to release old patterns, to open our hearts, and start to trust that *everything* is possible! This is our true journey, the healing for which we took birth.

Thank you, Mytrae, for writing this book to help us on the path.

Barbara Brodsky
Founding teacher of Deep Spring Center, Ann Arbor, MI
http://cosmichealingmeditation.com   http://deepspring.org
Author of *Cosmic Healing: A Spiritual Journey
with Aaron and John of God*

To the Blessed Entities of Light and Love
at the Casa de Dom Inácio
who have given me healing, gifts, and miracles
beyond what I could dream up for myself

and

to João Teixeira de Faria or "John of God"
for his extraordinary dedication and mission in this lifetime

ACKNOWLEDGMENTS

I AM DEEPLY GRATEFUL to several people who helped create this book.

To Beverly Bellinger, original inspirer, for persisting to help me realize that this guide could be useful to others.

To the beautiful people who traveled with me to the Casa, I have been honored by your trust. This book was written because of you.

I am so very grateful to many wonderful people who gave their time, love, and care to review the manuscript. Thank you for your hearts, generosity, and valuable feedback: Barbara Brodsky, Calvin Cates, Diego Coppola, Brant Cortright, Deb Court, Bob Dinga, David Lincoln King, Grainne McEntee, Yael Melamed, Shipra Narruhn, Greg Palma, Michael Quinn, Josie RavenWing, Ashley Rabun, Diana Rose, and Catherine Tucker.

Many thanks to my writing friends who read portions of the manuscript: David Fredrickson, Gina Genovese, Charlene Nevill, and Gabriella West.

And to dear friends, thank you for your friendship, encouragement, and support: Kerry Cadambi, Pam Alexander, Jane Hogan, and Barbara Rose Billings.

Thank you with all my heart.

John of God

> "I do not cure anybody. God heals,
> and in his infinite goodness permits
> the Entities to heal and console my brothers.
> I am merely an instrument in God's divine hands."
>
> —JOHN OF GOD

JOHN OF GOD, or João Teixeira de Faria, is a spiritual medium of extraordinary capacity. He channels evolved beings of Light and Love who heal people on multiple levels: physical, emotional, energetic, karmic, and spiritual.

Born in 1942 in a central Brazilian village, João was raised by his father, who was a tailor, and his mother, who ran a small hotel. João only attended a couple of grades of school. The poor family often went hungry, so he had to begin work at a very young age.

When he was nine, his psychic gifts revealed themselves while he was visiting family in another town. He predicted a huge storm and convinced his family to move to a different house. Indeed, shortly thereafter, a storm hurled through the town, destroying several homes, but not the one in which João and his family took refuge.

João left home at twelve or thirteen to make his way in the world. Doing various trade jobs and manual labor, he moved from village to town, finding work as he could. He often went hungry in his young, tender years.

At sixteen, he was traveling between towns and stopped by a stream in a forest one day. He hadn't eaten for a couple of days. A beautiful woman appeared and conversed with him at length. So taken was he by her appearance and what she said that he returned to the same place the next day. A brilliant light illuminated where she had sat, and her voice directed him to go to the Spiritist center in a town nearby. He didn't understand her message but did as she said, hoping he'd get a meal. Much later, he realized she was St. Rita of Cassia.

When he arrived at the Spiritist center, he "fell unconscious." When he came to, the director of the center told João that he had incorporated (channeled) the Entity of King Solomon, performed amazing surgeries, and healed several people. João, in complete disbelief, apologized for fainting because he hadn't eaten in a couple of days. The director went on to say that João, in his healing state, had said he'd return the next day. The director invited him to sleep at his home that night, which João willingly accepted, for he knew he'd get a meal. The next morning, João filled his stomach to capacity, unsure when his next meal would be, and nervously accompanied the director to the center. Once again, he "fell unconscious" and when he came to, he was told he had healed tens of people.

Needless to say, it took the adolescent João some time to accept the enormity and scope of his otherworldly gift and life mission. He was channeling a group of highly evolved beings, referred to as Entities. With St. Ignatius de Loyola at the helm, the group consists of saints, masters, doctors, and surgeons who have passed and want to work through him to heal people. In healing others, they themselves evolve. The Entities of Casa de Dom Inácio include St. Francis of Assisi, St. Francis Xavier, and St. Rita of Cassia. Several of them, like Dr. Augusto de Almeida, Dr. Oswaldo Cruz, and Dr. José Valdevino, were doctors and surgeons in their recent earth incarnations.

These Entities, over several months, instructed and guided Medium João in understanding his life purpose and how to work with them. Realizing that João was no ordinary medium, the director and people at the center wholeheartedly supported him.

For several years, Medium João traveled across Brazil healing hundreds of people, supported by volunteers. The name João de Deus, or John of God, was not one that he chose for himself; instead it was fondly given to him by the people he encountered. He has faced severe resistance from the religious and medical establishments, who were threatened by his gifts and had him imprisoned numerous times.

When Brazil's government became a military power in 1962, Medium João found refuge with the army as a tailor. But his healing gifts were soon discovered, and he found grateful patrons and protectors in high places. For the nine years that Brazil was under a dictatorship, Medium João was protected from persecution.

In 1978, the Entities told him to expand his work to reach more people. Chico Xavier, Brazil's extraordinary psychographic medium who channeled over four hundred books, guided Medium João to Abadiania, a small town in Goiania, the province where he was born. There, over more than thirty years, his work has grown from healing under a tree to a spiritual hospital, Casa de Dom Inácio, with several buildings, healing and treatment rooms, a bookstore, and a pharmacy.

Finally, Medium João had found a home for his family and healing work, and he is now protected by Brazilian authorities, who recognize and honor his incredible gifts to them and humanity. The Casa de Dom Inácio, House of St. Ignatius, received its name from and is directed by the patron saint and leading Entity behind John of God's work. The spiritual hospital serves as a training ground for thousands of Entities, who evolve through service. They work in teams on people, healing in every way, including past-life karma, shifting awareness and perspective, and raising energetic vibrations.

Medium João is a full-trance medium, which means that he leaves his body completely, enabling a very pure channel without ego interference through which the channeled Entity can work. Medium João has no recollection of what takes place while he is incorporated.

Millions flock to John of God, now in his seventies, from Brazil, USA, Europe, and all over the world for healing. All his healing is offered for free. In his regular life as a man, he supports himself and his family as an astute businessman. He remains humble, grateful, and most unpretentious about his amazing gifts. ⟨logo a march⟩

To learn more about *John of God*, the Casa de Dom Inácio, and the Entities, read John of God and visit www.friendsofthecasa. info and www.abadianiaportal.com.

My Healing Journey

"Come, come, whoever you are,
Wanderer, worshiper, lover of leaving.
It doesn't matter.
Ours is not a caravan of despair.
Come, even if you have broken your vows
a thousand times.
Come, yet again, come, come."

—RUMI

THREE DREAMS IN early 2009, just after I was licensed as a psychotherapist, marked the beginning of my journey to John of God.

My first dream:

I'm in another realm. I know it because of ethereal music I hear played by instruments not from this world, with sounds and frequencies I've never heard before. My ears open to a frequency of sound from another dimension.

I'm in a large enclosed space, its walls made of a non-solid yet solid material, and without a ceiling. There are thirty to forty other beings from various dimensions, some taller than humans, some shorter, and some our height. Some even look different. All walk or stand, conversing in small groups with dignity and presence. There is an air of sanctity, solemnity, and purpose to this gathering.

It is my initiation. It is a magnificent honor to join this group, one beyond my wildest dreams.

It is about music. I am to be initiated into something connected with music. All that I know presently about music is nothing compared with what I'm going to learn. It is completely new and different. These beings are here to teach me, show me, guide me.

My second dream:

My body feels and looks like a mountain range, with curves and undulations of warm brown skin. I hear a message: "You are about to go through something. It is a purification. It will feel like golden light passing through you. You will come out the other side."

I have an experience of golden light slowly passing through my entire body, from head to toe.

My third dream:

I am lying on my back. There are beings above me. They are working on my chest with a piece of incredibly complex and intricate equipment, about six inches square. Spindles and needles, wheels and cranks—the terms sound heavy and dense, yet this instrument is made of the finest, strongest, most delicate materials. In comparison, a clock mechanism seems like it's from the dinosaur age, and a steel scalpel cruder than a caveman's club.

The beings use the equipment to work on me. Things are being extracted from me. The equipment is first a few inches above my chest, then enters my chest, then is removed and hovers above my chest. The work is complete. It's as though . . . as though they are performing surgery on me! It's not physical surgery, like on my organs, muscles, or bones, but . . . energetic . . . psychic!

I woke with a start. What *was* that? I could still feel the equipment above me, so real, as if it was happening in actual time. Surgery? Psychic surgery? What *is* that? Is there such a thing as psychic surgery?

Googling for "psychic surgery" brought up Philippine healers about whom I was skeptical. Yet my dream experience had been so refined and sophisticated.

* * *

A few months later, Brant, my very healthy partner, suddenly developed a health issue. The best doctors ran their most advanced tests but couldn't diagnose him. He recalled hearing about John of God from one of his students at the graduate school where he teaches psychology. He was both open to and wary of energy healers, having heard lots of stories of false promises.

But we were desperate. Western medicine didn't have any solutions for Brant, and we needed to look outside that paradigm.

When he asked me what I thought about John of God, I checked out a few sites online. My healing had been through psychotherapy and related holistic modalities, and I hadn't worked with energy healers. I had no context for spiritual healing, yet something about John of God rang true. I encouraged him to go.

Brant went to Abadiania for a week and was blown away by the energy at the Casa. He's had a deep spiritual path for forty years, and his work integrates spirituality and psychology. He's visited ashrams in India and explored many spiritual states. Yet, when we Skyped, he said, "I feel incredible here. I don't need to take my medication. I've never experienced anything like it. The energy practically takes the roof off the building! You *have* to come here!"

I was so excited for him, that he'd found a healing way. We decided to go there together that December.

* * *

A series of events catapulted me toward a visit to John of God sooner.

A homeless person slept in my car overnight. I had left my car windows open one night when I parked on a street near Haight-Ashbury, a San Francisco neighborhood where homeless people abound.

A couple days later, I felt pinpricks all over my body, as though I was pricked by a thousand needles. Soon, I had horrific crawling sensations, as though a hundred tiny worms inhabited my body, even inside my nose, eyes, and ears. I was horrified and terrified, as though I'd been flung into a pit of snakes. I felt as though my life had turned upside down and inside out.

Thinking it might be Lyme, a practitioner prescribed

antibiotics and sleeping pills, and had me tested for the disease. I approached healing on multiple fronts: cleansing, diet, herbs, supplements, and homeopathy. I plastered myself with clay and soaked in Dead Sea salt water. I toned and chanted. I did my inner work, had intuitive readings, and explored my emotional relationship to being a leper. I wrote to Mother Meera in Germany, asking for her blessings and healing Light. I sent my picture to John of God for distance healing.

My partner, Brant, was a calming and soothing presence amid my panic and chaos. Despite my horror and fear, I also experienced incredible streams of Divine Light entering me, which, along with Mother Meera's radiant picture, were a spiritual lifeline.

One day, covered with Dead Sea clay, I knew I needed to go to John of God. While making preparations, I felt as though my way was being cleared—everything fell into place incredibly smoothly, in contrast to the chaos of my life. Even though I was very late in applying for my visa at the Brazilian consulate, the woman made a special concession for me since I was visiting John of God.

My distance healing guide emailed to say she took my picture to John of God *on the same day I knew I needed to go*! The Entity Dr. Augusto had said, "Tell all of these people that if they are ever able to come here they should come!"

The day before I left for Brazil, my landlady banged on my door and shouted, "Fire! Fire! Get out!" I rushed outside to see a fire blazing in three homes, firemen hosing the buildings, and a couple hundred people who'd gathered to watch. Fortunately, my things were safe, even though my landlady's home above me was burned and waterlogged.

My body. My car. My home. My three physical foundations were being attacked. *What next?*

Those six weeks had cracked me wide open. I flew to Brasilia, desperate and completely open to whatever I would receive at the Casa de Dom Inácio. I felt ready to release whatever needed to be released and prepare for the life that was in store for me.

Catherine Tucker of Pousada Luz Divina arranged for a taxi to meet me at Brasilia airport, and it was a lovely ride through the countryside's gently rolling green hills. The brightly colored, simple buildings and lush, tropical foliage reminded me of India.

Mateus, the friendly taxi driver, regaled me with stories of amazing healings. People being healed of cancer, their hearing restored, being able to walk after years in a wheelchair. Could this really be true? Would I be healed too?

Abadiania was a small, unpretentious town. The people looked unhurried and friendly. I stayed at Pousada Luz Divina, a charming inn with a beautiful garden and lovely people. It was a perfect place to heal.

I hired a local guide who showed me around the Casa, where I felt a deep sense of comfort. At my first Casa session, my guide translated my requests: "Please heal me of parasites. Please heal my emotional trauma. Please guide me in my healing work."

I went in the second time line, since I had had a distance healing. My guide said, "Look in the Entity's eyes. If he puts out his hand, put yours in it." The Entity smiled at and nodded to me. "I will help you. Sit in my Current."

I was hugely relieved to hear his words. During the three hours of Current, the meditation and healing session, I felt physically uncomfortable and agitated, needing to wiggle my restless legs—unusual, for I'm a long-time meditator. I felt energies squirming out through my soles.

In two days, my crawling sensations stopped, to my huge relief. My pinpricks alternated between intensifying and reducing by seventy-five percent. I stopped my sleeping medication. I had powerful dreams of beings healing and working with me. And dreams of being terrified while streams of light extended toward me with the instruction, "Hold on to the light." I did. I kept hearing "Fatima." I later realized that Fatima is another name for Mother Mary. The Divine Feminine seemed to be on loudspeakers while I was at the Casa—I felt Her everywhere, saw Her everywhere—powerfully, strongly, and deeply.

I asked my guide about my intensified pinpricks and he said, "You receive a spiritual healing when you're here. Some things happen instantly, but often, since the cause is worked on, the symptoms take time to be released through your energetic, emotional, and physical bodies. As your symptoms are working out of your field, it can seem like they're increasing."

I had invisible surgery, which was incredible and came with some physical discomfort. I had a pounding headache, slept a lot, and had amazing visions. I felt held, taken care of, and known on every level.

At the interfaith service on Sunday where we sang hymns and read prayers, I cried quietly, feeling a love beyond anything I've ever experienced. As I left, an incredible Love entered my heart—exalted, powerful, and divine. It was a Love not of this world. It entered my deepest places, my core. Sitting on a bench at the outlook, I felt the Love cradle the part of me that feels unlovable, like a leper, an outcast. This absolutely unconditional Love pierced, engulfed, and enveloped my deepest wounding. *I am loved simply for who I am. I don't have to do anything to be loved.* I sat for an hour, dissolved in sobs, opening to and receiving this incredible Love.

My second week was about emotional healing, and I kept feeling the Love. The Entities communicated through visions, dreams, messages, and knowings. It was wonderful to talk with other pousada guests, share experiences, learn about Spiritism and the extraordinary healing paradigm channeled by John of God.

At the waterfall, I had a vision of myself standing above it as my negative emotions spewed out of me. I flung them out and away, and they transformed into beautiful flowers that sprang out into the world. I heard again and again, "You are healed, child. You are healed."

Incredibly moved and filled with gratitude for all that I'd received, I asked during a crystal bed session, one of the healing modalities at the Casa, "Please show me how I may serve." Instantly, I saw a movie of me bringing people wearing white clothes to the Casa. "Me?!" I doubted, feeling so incapable of that.

* * *

Back in San Francisco, I learned that my Lyme test results were positive. I had made an appointment with Dr. Steve Harris, a holistic Lyme specialist, before leaving for Brazil. He said, "With your car, body, and house being hit, it was probably a psychic attack." I hadn't expected such a diagnosis from a medical doctor! "Your positive Lyme tests don't mean anything. You can be Lyme positive and not have any symptoms. You have two to three Lyme co-infections, which we'll treat with herbs. Continue your cleansing and diet. Go do your emotional work. You're going to be fine. I have several clients who've been to John of God. Stop the antibiotics when you go to John of God in December. Take these herbs until your symptoms stop for three months, then stop them too. You don't need to see me again."

I was blown away by his clean bill of health!

I also went to the first practitioner who wanted to see me after the Lyme test results were in. She said, "You can stop the antibiotics in a couple of months. And you don't have to come back and see me again."

Wow! Two doctors confirmed the same thing: I was healed! Moreover, I *felt* healed, and that it was only a question of time before I was completely well.

After eighteen months, my symptoms completely stopped and have never returned, except very occasionally and mildly when there's an eclipse or a super moon.

On my third trip to the Casa, while sitting in Current, I felt ready to ask for permission to bring people to the Casa. I heard the Entities chuckle and communicate in the way they do, "We told you the first time!"

I took my first group in June 2012. Nine amazing people who received beautiful healings. Now, I take groups, which fills me with profound joy, wonder, gratitude, and fun. Every time I go, I experience extraordinary Love and healing, and I am so taken care of as a guide. I feel deeply blessed and honored to do this work.

In spring 2013 my partner, Brant, was also completely healed.

I feel completely transformed since my first visit in August 2009. My work as a psychotherapist has changed. My work has become more spiritual, as I am much more intuitive. I'm increasingly connected to the Entities' guidance, as well as that of my guides and angels. They teach me how to work with Light, energy, and vibration.

The Entities help me work more quickly and efficiently with challenging situations. Challenges are gifts, which I've learned to discover by shifting what's within me. And when I've no idea how to resolve a situation or relationship, I ask for and surrender to the Entities' guidance, and it gets resolved or healed in a way that is nothing short of miraculous.

I can ask for anything if I'm aligned with and ready to receive it. There's usually growth involved—letting go of a smaller way of being and opening to a larger one. I've received incredible gifts, like being able to play the piano again (something very precious to me) after decades, reconciliation with estranged family, buying a magical home among redwoods, opportunities and professional contacts that materialize out of the ether, and wonderful friends and community.

The Entities help, heal, and teach me in every way. Almost every aspect of my life has changed, and I trust that even more will evolve in good time. My life has so much more play, joy, laughter, and ease. I live an almost fearless life instead of being filled with fear, the way I used to live. I feel so much joy, gratitude, and creativity. I feel as though I've stepped into life's magic, which I knew as a child, yet lost as I became an adult. The magic of being. The amazing power of Love. And the incredible energy of Light.

With deep gratitude and joy, I share my story and this book with you.

Happy journey and blessings!

The Call

"We have been called to heal wounds,
to unite what has fallen apart,
and to bring home those who have lost their way."

—St. Francis of Assisi

PEOPLE ARE CALLED to the Casa de Dom Inácio.
By pain or by love.

You may be called by physical sickness or disease. By mental health issues. By grief over losing someone or something very precious. By reaching the very desperate end of what you know, and seeking something beyond that. Or something else. You may be facing something so painful and frustrating and challenging, which those around you, including health professionals, can't help you with, that you consider or feel like going to Brazil to see John of God.

Or you may go for love. Hearing about him and the Entities may stir your heart and soul. You may see his face in your dreams, prayers, or meditation. You may go to accompany someone you love. You may suddenly start hearing about him. You may read a book or see a video about him. Something about the energy when someone speaks about him or you see him in a video sets your cells and soul vibrating, like a tuning fork. You just feel guided to go.

You may have heard about him for years and always meant to go. It feels right. You've just been waiting for the right time. Suddenly one day, you hear the Call. From within yourself, your guides, or from someone else. And you know you're going. Soon. You sit back to wait and see how it will all unfold.

It happens. Just like that.

Suddenly, one day, you find yourself looking at airline ticket prices, visa information, or for a guide to help you travel to a foreign country with even more foreign experiences, such as invisible surgery and crystal baths and beings who heal from the other side of the veil.

Then your doubts and skepticism assail you.

"What am I doing?"

"This is crazy!"

"How can this possibly help me?!"

Still, you find yourself reading about him on the Internet or in a book, and the prospect of going there keeps popping into your mind or tugging at your heart. Some part of you is curious. Fascinated.

Because the question "What if . . . ?" lurks in your heart.

You can't believe that you're thinking of going, but you find yourself unable to resist the urge to make preparations, as if you have already decided to go.

You've heard the Call. And you're responding. Once you hear it, it may take a while for the rest of you to catch up!

Once you respond, it all works out at the right time. When? How? With or without money. Even when it is physically challenging to travel.

Once you respond to the Call, the Entities help you get to Abadiania, Brazil.

What Can I Expect?

"For those who believe, no proof is necessary.
For those who disbelieve, no amount of proof is sufficient."
—St. Ignatius de Loyola

Can I expect a miracle?

YES. ABSOLUTELY. THOUSANDS of people have received miraculous healings. People have been healed from cancer and all kinds of diseases. People in wheelchairs or on crutches have become able to walk. People who can't see or hear have their vision or hearing restored. People with mental illness are cured after a single visit.

Having said that, your miracle may not look exactly like what you'd expect.

- ◆ Healing is a process, not an event.

◆ You don't get what you want—you get what you need! You may need to heal another area or areas of your life first.

◆ Your healing may be instantaneous or rapid. More often, though, it's a series of shifts and transformations. The Entities often heal in layers, each layer transforming as necessary and as you're ready.

◆ Your challenge could well be an opportunity to grow. People who don't receive instant physical healing often have shifts in other parts of their life. You'll frequently hear people say, "My illness brought me here, but even though I still have _____, I've received so much in other areas of my life. I now see how my _____ is an incredible gift. I've transformed in so many ways. I would never have discovered all that without _____."

◆ What you're dealing with might be something you've come into this life to experience. It may be a soul contract or lesson you set up. And your soul's goal, no matter how difficult and challenging, is not to eradicate the challenge but to evolve because of and through it.

◆ Your whole being receives healing, something that you cannot direct or have control over. Healing is not compartmentalized to certain aspects of yourself. You may think you have only physical issues or are only going for your spiritual work, but all of you receives healing.

◆ Very occasionally, based on your karma, the Entities
may say that they cannot help you. If it is your karma
to experience something, they cannot change things
or intervene. If this is the case, they will let you know.

What's a spiritual hospital?

The Casa de Dom Inácio is referred to as a spiritual hospital
because it helps you connect to your spiritual nature. It is a
hospital for your soul.

As Pierre Teilhard de Chardin said, "We are not human
beings having a spiritual experience; we are spiritual beings
having a human experience." We are magnificent beings
of Love, Wisdom, Beauty, Truth, Power, Light, and much
more. We incarnate as human beings to experience life so we
can evolve as souls. Having an ego and personality naturally
distances us from our Higher Self, our soul.

Going to the Casa helps you connect more deeply with
your spiritual nature. It also helps you connect with the Divine,
God, Goddess, Source, Spirit, or whichever term you use for
the Sacred and Transcendent. When you open to who you
are as a soul and to the Transcendent, Grace, Love, and Light
enter you. This alone can clear and heal.

Many people who visit the Casa experience unconditional
Love, exalted beings, high vibrations, and Light in their bodies
and energy fields.

Visiting the Casa is a 24/7 experience

Going to the Casa is like going on a spiritual healing retreat.

It's a 24/7 experience. You're being worked on not only on
Casa days, in surgery, or under the crystal bed, but *all the time*!

As mentioned earlier, work on you begins once you decide to visit the Casa; it intensifies while you're there.

Each moment is a wonderful opportunity to be with, process, shift, and let go of what you need to heal and evolve.

You may think you receive healing only while the Casa's in session or while receiving specific treatments, but if you tune in to yourself in silence, reflection, or meditation, you discover that a lot more is going on.

Socializing is a great way to share, validate, and learn from your experiences and make wonderful connections, but watch out for it becoming a distraction. The same applies for reading, being online, and engaging in any other activity. Take full advantage of the short time you're there; the more you can go inward, stay silent, and become aware, the more you participate, shift, and transform.

A lot of the work is done at night when your resistance and defenses are down. You may have vivid or significant dreams, some of which you understand and some that will make sense later. Make note of them! You might find yourself awake in the early hours of the morning, refreshed even after a few hours of sleep. Or that it's hard to sleep deeply.

Every moment is a learning, growing, and healing opportunity. There are teams of Entities with you, working on you. So much incredible guidance and transformation is at hand just for you.

Take advantage of it!

Why are there so many rules?

All the rules or protocols are prescribed by the Entities for your optimum healing.

The more closely you follow the rules, the more you participate and give the Entities the best opportunity to work on you.

Think of protocols as a handshake—this is what the Entities ask you to do so they can best help you. For instance, wearing white clothes on Casa days enables them to see your spiritual aura clearly. And the post-surgery instructions and herbs help the Entities best work with you. It's not unlike having a physical surgery in a regular hospital, after which your surgeon asks you to restrict certain activities or stick to a particular diet.

If you have any resistance about the protocols, you may want to explore whether you have a similar response to rules in general. It could lead to some deeper self-awareness.

You may hear a few interpretations of the rules based on whom you talk with. Make sure to talk with a guide or Casa volunteer to get an accurate interpretation.

Your own guidance does *not* override the Entity's prescription for you! The Entities state that if you choose not to follow the protocols, they're not responsible for your healing.

Please consult the *Official Casa Guide* for all Casa protocols and terminology.

Hmmm . . . I'm skeptical

Stay skeptical. Don't change a thing!

You don't have to believe or buy into anything. Bring your doubts and ambivalence and skepticism along on your journey. Your mind is an essential part of you—all your questions and doubts are valid. When encountering a paradigm so different from your reality, how could you not have questions, doubts, and skepticism?

Let your own experience be your guide. You're not supposed to and don't have to believe anything or have faith to visit John of God.

John of God and the Casa de Dom Inácio are spiritual but not religious. John of God doesn't claim formal association with any religion or tradition. He was raised Catholic, so while there are Catholic images and figurines at the Casa, he chooses not to identify with it. The same with being a Spiritist—even though his work is within the Spiritist tradition, he doesn't claim to be one. Even on the egoic and personality levels, John of God doesn't claim to be enlightened or a healer. In his words, "I do not heal; God is the one who heals."

The Casa de Dom Inácio is nondenominational and is open to everyone regardless of your religious or nonreligious background. It has no management or authorities. Everything that happens there is created, managed, and guided by the Entities.

While there, you're not pressured or indoctrinated or seduced to be part of the Casa or the Spiritist tradition. There are no followers or devotees of John of God, since there are no teachings other than what you receive from your own experience. All healing is free, except herbs, crystal bed sessions, and blessed water, which is the same cost as bottled water. There are no solicitations for donations. You are free to come and go as you please.

You receive what you receive while you're there. Nothing is expected or asked of you.

So bring your skepticism and curiosity and doubts along on your journey.

What Does Healing Look Like at the Casa?

"My phalange comprises not of ten,
nor a hundred, but thousands of Helping Spirits.
I am the one who reaches to the very depths
of the abyss to save a soul."
—DR. AUGUSTO DE ALMEIDA

Healing is holographic

HEALING AT THE Casa is holographic. That means that the Entities see you as a hologram, as a whole being with several interconnected aspects or layers: spiritual, emotional, physical, mental, energetic, karmic, soul purpose, and past lives. They know every aspect of you and your life, including relationships, family, work, gifts and talents, financial, creativity etc., and want to help you heal and evolve.

The Entities also know all about your soul's journey, purpose, and contracts. They assist your soul in its highest purpose. You came into this life with certain contracts and to learn certain lessons through various situations and relationships. They help you with every part of it. They help you become aligned, harmonious, and connected to all that you are.

Healing often shows up as what you
need, not what you want.

Sometimes people want only physical healing or spiritual growth. But holographic healing is about the whole. If you only want physical healing, it's likely connected to something that's not about your body, but about your emotional state, approach to life, relationships, or past-life karma. It could well be that you need to learn or shift something outside of your illness. Likewise, if you focus only on your spirituality and ignore your sick body, the Entities begin with the physical. Your body is an integral part of who you are. Wholeness is including and integrating all aspects of your being.

A different paradigm

The Entities' healing is of a completely different paradigm than what you may be familiar with. They heal through exalted vibrations of Light and Love.

Barbara Brodsky's book *Cosmic Healing* gives a wonderful account of their healing, as narrated by Aaron, her personal Entity.

Clearing attachments

Almost everyone who goes to the Casa has attachments, spirits who've attached themselves to us. The Entities are the best clearers of unwanted attachments.

In the Spiritist tradition, physical or mental illness is often attributed to a being or beings connected to a person. These beings could be a soul in limbo, a relative who has passed, a spirit randomly picked up, or a negative entity. These beings, for whatever reason, are lost or not connected to the Light. Usually we have a corresponding vibrational "hook," like an emotion or belief, which attracts and links them to us.

The Entities clear these attachments from us and transport them to the Light. This is another reason people instantly feel better when visiting the Casa.

Healing and growth

Healing and growth are two sides of a single coin.

If this is your first time, you're most likely going to the Casa for healing. When you heal some part of yourself, it creates space for something new to enter your life.

For instance, if you have a physical illness such as cancer, its roots may lie in something emotional like anger or fear, a broken or closed heart, a self-limiting belief, or not being aligned with your soul purpose. Physical illness is often a dire call from your body that you're not paying attention to something essential. It's also a sign that you're ready to grow out of a smaller way of being. Your body's message may be as simple as needing to give yourself more rest, better nourishment, and exercise. It might be connected with a way you are in the world, like how you are in relationships, work, letting go of a smaller way of being, or opening more to your authentic or spiritual nature. It might even be as obscure and complex as being ready to resolve some past-life karma.

These are some questions and issues that will come up as a part of your healing. Going to the Casa to heal propels you to grow in ways you don't yet know.

Alternatively, you may be going to the Casa to grow and transform in a particular area. For instance, you may want to connect more spiritually, receive guidance and clarity about your work or life purpose, have a family, find a loving relationship, or develop supportive, meaningful relationships and community. When you want to grow, you know you need to let go of a smaller way of being or an identity you're outgrowing. You know you're ready for your next phase of expansion.

Healing and growth are reciprocal. As you heal, you may find yourself growing in an area of your life. And as you grow, you may heal and transform.

Healing is a process, not an event

Going to the Casa is a process. Everything about it is. The more you understand and attune to your process, the more you receive.

Your healing is a process. It's *not* a final, discrete, and permanent state or event.

And, *you* are a process. You are *in* process. Of healing and growth and evolution.

When you latch on to an idea of a fixed state of health or identity, you lose so much more that's waiting for you. When you're fixed about something, you shut out so much. Your healing may need you to look at a completely different area than where you think the issue lies. It's an opportunity to be curious. What will your healing look like?

Your process is like a sequence of stepping stones. Each choice, each decision you make, carries you to a new place. From there, you have a completely new set of choices.

You have choices and make choices every moment. Tuning in to your choices and how you make choices is a great way to stay open, fresh, curious, and inviting.

Some ways to begin:

◆ What are you choosing?

◆ On what basis do you choose?

◆ What beliefs, assumptions, and feelings inform or compel you to choose this?

◆ Is there space for other possibilities?

◆ What else is possible?

◆ Are there other ways you haven't tried?

◆ What would it be like, and how would you feel, if you were to do something different?

Healing is a series of shifts

When you meet people at the Casa, you will talk with many who are visiting for the nth time. You will hear people say that each time, a new level has been healed.

Going to John of God is not like going to a magician who waves a magic wand. Sometimes that happens, and those are the miraculous, instantaneous healings. You may well have that. More often, it's a gradual series of shifts.

The Entities heal by doing fifty percent of the work, and you're expected to do the other fifty percent. This is crucial to remember. You can't sit back and expect them to do everything. Your participation is critical (that's part of what this book helps you with).

Each time you visit, you're a little more ready to release what you need to. You've grown a little more. You're a little further along on your journey.

The Entities work with you where you are each time you visit. Very gently, effectively, and with incredible compassion, nuance, and understanding. They know things take time to work out. Often there's emotional, spiritual, and karmic work to be done; knots to be untied, relationships to be worked out and worked through. All of this takes time.

So much of your healing is your growth.

And this simply cannot be rushed. They definitely help you with it. But they're not going to do it for you. That's *your* work.

The Entities go as fast as you're able to go.

Why Should I Prepare?

"Before anything else,
preparation is the key to success."
—ALEXANDER GRAHAM BELL

PREPARING TO VISIT the Casa de Dom Inácio helps you get the most out of your stay there. It's a wonderful way to begin your process before you visit the Casa. Your preparation:

◆ Allows you to begin your healing before you get on the plane. You hit the ground running when you arrive. When you prepare beforehand, you extend the duration of your journey.

◆ Builds your capacity to work while you're in Abadiania. Inner work is very much like a muscle. The more you do it, the more you can do. When you begin before you go, you maximize how much you can clear, release, and shift while you are there.

You maximize how much you can receive from the Entities.

◆ Strengthens your connection with the Entities. The moment you decide to go to the Casa, the Entities begin working with you. Since your healing is participatory, the more you work on yourself, the more the Entities work with you.

◆ Widens your channels of invitation and receptivity to the Entities. You begin learning how to work with the Entities before you go—you may notice shifts and changes. Your dreams may intensify. The Entities want to help you heal and grow. They want to give you all that you can receive. You may be more open to receive in some areas than others. Your preparation tills the soil of yourself.

◆ Opens the parts of you that are closed, constricted, hard, or wounded (aka blocks); these parts need the rain of your attention, even if you don't know what to do with them. They soften, even if only by your awareness and willingness to look at and be with them.

◆ You may not imagine that you can do and gain more with your gifts and capacities. Simply wanting more for yourself prepares you to open in ways you can't imagine.

◆ You may be asking some essential questions, such as:

  ◈ Who am I?

- Why am I here?

- What am I meant to do in my life?

- What has my life been about?

◆ You might find your time well spent in beginning your reflection on such questions before you visit.

Types of preparation

There are two types of preparation.

1. Logistics

You decide when to go, where to stay, and whom to select as a guide, if you're using one. You book tickets, make lists, clear your calendars, and prepare for the trip. These are all essential.

You may also want and try to understand everything about the Casa, learn how the healing happens, and understand its structure. There's a lot of information you can get from books and videos.

The chapter on logistics gives you more information about this.

Other excellent resources for logistical preparation are:

◆ *John of God* by Heather Cumming and Karen Leffler

◆ http://www.abadianiaportal.com, a comprehensive website on visiting Abadiania and the Casa.

◆ http://www.friendsofthecasa.info, a website that offers information and an official guide to visiting the Casa.

2. Your spiritual and emotional preparation

Preparing for the Casa is different from preparing for a vacation. It's outside the bounds of the religion and spirituality and modes of healing you know, no matter how "out there" you've traveled.

The best way to prepare is with your heart, being, and soul. Prepare to open and be willing to do something completely outside your frame of reference. Prepare to look outside what you know to be true.

It's getting ready to shift big stuff. It's becoming willing to sit with difficult questions, feelings, and issues. It's preparing to dive into old, old stuff, even things that happened long ago and from which you may have already done much healing.

When you decide to go, you're saying, "I'm ready to open to what I don't know. I'm ready to transform. Now." Some live life in this way. For others, it's the scariest thing in the world to step into the unknown.

The best kind of preparation is a leap of faith where what you commit to is to show up for yourself. Fully. Completely. All of you. And hope and trust that you'll be caught, held, and healed by something or someone larger than yourself.

How Do I Prepare?

"Life is an unfoldment, and the further we travel
the more truth we can comprehend.
To understand the things that are at our door
is the best preparation for understanding
those that lie beyond."

——Hypatia

Set aside time

SET ASIDE TIME to reflect and meditate in the weeks or days before your visit to the Casa. The Entities begin working with you once you decide to go, so you may feel their presence and guidance.

Preparing for your healing journey is so important. There is the possibility for so much—healing, growth, shifts, openings, miracles, and transformation. Like a marathon runner, the more you prepare or open to surrender, the more you receive.

Set aside time to emotionally and spiritually prepare. If the questions in this book resonate with you, sit with, reflect upon, and answer them.

Also, prepare for your return. Take care of routine things that you might need to do for a month or so after you return. Clear as much space as you can, reducing activities and commitments to a minimum. Prepare to be as internal as your life allows after you return. You may undergo a deep shift, and it can be very beneficial to have lots of alone time to process, integrate, and allow what's unfolding and transforming to take root in you.

Why am I going?

Spend some time reflecting on why you're going. Distill your intention until it's pure and simple. Get really clear.

Here are some questions to reflect on to help you get clear:

◆ Why am I going?

◆ What is this journey about for me?

◆ Why now?

◆ What do I truly want to change?

◆ And why?

◆ Who would I be if I changed?

◆ How would I feel if I changed?

◆ What will all that change mean for me?

◆ Is this change within myself or outside myself?

◆ Is the reason I'm going responsible for making me

unhappy and stressed, or might there be a deeper reason I don't know about, am afraid to face, or cannot yet feel?

Review your life

What do you want healing on?

What part of yourself or your life do you want to grow and transform?

Make a list of all the areas of your life. Here are some areas to help you get started. Perhaps you have a few more?

◆ Physical

◆ Emotional

◆ Energetic and psychic

◆ Spiritual

◆ Relationships

◆ Work / career / creativity / life purpose

◆ Money and material resources

Stay open!

Staying open is one of the most important ways in which to prepare. Be open to all your experiences: thoughts, emotions, sensations, intuition, energy, and dreams. Stay open to your judgments, skepticism, doubts, criticism, negative emotions, and resistance. Stay open to receiving in every obvious and subtle way. Stay open to shifts in perspective and aha moments. Stay open to images, messages, knowings, and guidance you receive.

Stay open to every moment and interaction. There are teachings and lessons everywhere and in everything.

Everything that comes up is an opportunity to shift something. To grow. To heal.

Stay open like a child. Take your inner child along with you.

Watch and listen for what you don't yet know

At the Casa, healing and growth often lie outside of what you know. And in a completely different area. When you think you know, you create a lid or crust-like limitation around yourself and your world. When you stay open to what you don't yet know, you're receptive.

Physical illness, even the most severe diagnosis, is an opportunity to heal or shift something. It could be emotional healing by opening to love or living from joy and creativity. It could be spiritual healing by reconnecting in a new way with the Divine and your divinity.

Try holding what's most challenging, like your physical illness or an impossible relationship, as an opportunity to look around, outside of, and beyond it. The gifts of your challenges often lie in dark, untouched, and forgotten places.

For instance, you may go for physical healing yet receive a healing of your heart or discover your life purpose. A man goes to heal his cancer and finds he has healed after resolving a difficult relationship. Another person's depression lifts after she lets go of her deceased mother. Healing at the Casa often shows up in a completely different area than where you expect it.

Once you decide to go, watch, listen, dream, and open to sensing and intuiting.

◆ Watch who and what comes into your life or says something that speaks or resonates with you.

◆ Observe and note synchronicities.

◆ When you meditate, be open to receiving messages, images, or fantasies. Even words or phrases that feel like they "don't come from you."

◆ Look and listen for feelings, ideas, beliefs, perspectives that seem like they're broader, wider, more expansive than what you normally believe.

◆ Most importantly and especially, be open to what might feel beyond and outside your normal sphere of experience. Even and especially if you don't understand or believe. You might have experiences or messages that can seem "out there," "wild," or just "don't make sense." Simply write them down or make note of them. Often, you might understand them weeks, months, even years later!

◆ Many people find their intuition and psychic capacities open up at the Casa. This is because it's a safe place where these can flourish and open. They're also ways the Entities communicate with you. You might discover your gifts of clairaudience, clairsentience, claircognizance, and clairvoyance. So listen to those voices and remember those images, sensations, and knowings that "tell you things" or give you information!

How to Make
Your Requests

"Hope has two beautiful daughters;
their names are Anger and Courage.
Anger at the way things are,
and Courage to see that they do not remain as they are."

—St. Augustine of Hippo

Beginning your process

BEGIN AS SOON as you know you're going.

Get a piece of paper and pen, your smartphone, or your laptop/tablet and make a list of any and all of your requests.

Better still, get a notebook that you assign just for your journey to John of God. You will travel such a distance that you may want a journal of all you experience on your healing journey. You may want to look back and read how you got "here" from "there."

Begin by beginning. Write down what you know, then open up, letting your mind, ego, heart, and soul write. Don't worry about whether these musings are okay or too much or ridiculous or wild. They need to be. This is only the beginning of a process. You can edit it later.

It's easiest if your main reason for going is that you're physically sick. Because you know what you're asking for. You know it's your heart problem or cancer or eyesight. It's something you live with every day. You want to heal; you want to feel better. And you may be desperate; you may want relief with something that hinders your life, or it might be something you've just gotten used to and live around.

Preparing to visit the Casa is an opportunity to take stock of your life so you can receive all that you want from your visit. Think of everything you want now, at this time in your life. Think of all you've ever wanted over the course of your life, including things you've let go of because you couldn't imagine that they could ever happen or that you could ever heal, despite years of therapy and inner work. What have been your most difficult situations, traumas, or ruptured and broken relationships, even ones with people who've passed?

What are your deepest wounds? What's your worst pain? What beliefs do you have, such as "I don't deserve," "I'm not lovable," or "I'm not good enough"? Do you want to heal your depression, anxiety, trauma, mental health issues, or the way you exist in the world? Call forth your darkest feelings. These are uncomfortable questions, but often they are areas calling for healing or growth.

- ◆ Of what are you most afraid?

- What do you grieve? About what are you most sad?

- What is your deepest loss that still affects you?

- About what or with whom are you most angry?

- Who has hurt you?

- What traumatic experiences (physical and emotional) have you experienced?

- Whom or what do you hate?

- Of whom are you jealous?

- What are all the ways in which you make yourself small? If you could be all that you could be, who *would* you be? What do you not dare or dream to ask for?

- What do you absolutely not want anymore in your life? What do you feel done with and ready to let go of?

- If you can imagine having a different life, being differently in the world, only if . . . what would that be?

- If you could have everything you've ever wanted, what would that look like?

- What is the loudest call of your soul? What is the softest call of your soul?

Sit with these. Let them roll around you, inside you, as you go about your days and weeks. Keep writing them down as they occur to you.

You're not just creating a list; you're beginning your healing process.

Once you open up to asking, you might be surprised by the bonfire of desire and want burning within you. You may or may not be amazed by your hunger for what you want. There are no right or wrong questions and answers here—only what's authentic and true for you.

Why do I make requests?

"It's not okay to ask" is a message you may have heard growing up or have been socialized to believe. So you learn to restrain yourself, be polite, and to accept your life, situations, and relationships. You might even have been told that that's a spiritual way of being.

At the Casa, with the Entities, asking is necessary. Every time you go before the Entity, you can make up to three requests. Earlier, you read that the Entities do fifty percent of the work. The other fifty percent is yours. You can also go up to the Entity in complete surrender, without making any requests.

Even though the Entities know everything about you, requests are your participation in your healing process.

Why do you ask?

◆ You open up to hope.

◆ It's your part of the work. It shows the Entities your willingness and readiness to shift, to move to another level, to let go of a smaller way of feeling and being in the world.

◆ It's how you invite the Entities to work on you. They don't barge in, doing whatever they think, but wait for you to invite them. When you go to the Casa with your requests, whether you ask them or not, you hold them in your body, mind, heart, and soul. You hold the energy of what you most want in yourself. They see this holographically and work with where you are in that moment.

◆ The process of asking is your inner work. By engaging in it, you prepare yourself to receive from the Entities. When you ask, they direct an enormous amount of energy toward you. When you prepare, you amplify, take full advantage, and can make full use of what you receive. When you prepare, you're like a surfer waiting for a wave, ready to ride its swell when it comes your way.

◆ As part of your inner work, you may grapple with your limiting beliefs. You may come up against all your doubts and skepticism: "How is that possible?" "That can never change." "What hogwash!" "Boy, these people are really drinking the kool-aid!" You need to touch and know and feel your limiting beliefs and skepticism. They're along for the ride too! You can't discard, deny, or reject your skepticism. All of you gets to go to the Casa.

◆ When you ask, you open up to possibility.

Is it really okay to ask for physical things?

"Isn't that egotistical or vain?" people often ask.

Asking for physical things can be one of the hardest things for you to accept—that it's okay to ask! Especially for those of us who are "very spiritual." We think, "Oh, we're not supposed to ask for things for ourselves other than what's spiritual." But no. Think of the brazenly impossible, like a red convertible, a beautiful, comfortable home, or perfect health.

Ask! What does your ego crave? In fact, let your ego go wild and make a wish list. This is your chance to make a wish!

Only three requests?

"How can I squish my fifty-seven requests into three?!" people often exclaim.

It may be helpful to review your list and reduce them to ten. Which ones are absolutely essential? Select the three most important ones.

Review your list again and again—while driving, cooking, in the shower, on your meditation seat. Let your list be the background music to your life. As more requests come to you, add them to your list.

You will know which ones are most important. They call

out to you. Your eyes keep returning to them. You feel an ache in your chest as you think about them.

Then, categorize them:

◆ Physical

◆ Emotional

◆ Mental

◆ Spiritual

◆ Work, creativity, and life purpose

◆ Relationships

◆ Finances

◆ . . .

You can word them this way:

"Please heal my physical issues of A, B, C . . ."

"Please give me emotional and psychological healing."

"Please guide me in my spiritual growth."

"Please help me find my life purpose and work."

"Please help me find my soulmate."

"Please heal my _____."

"Please help me with _____."

"Please guide me with _____."

These are only suggestions. Ultimately, use wording that feels right to you.

You might find that you change and reword them a hundred times. Do. It's all part of your process. In this wording and rewording process, you're not only crafting your requests, you're building and honing the energy with which you hold them. The more strongly and deeply you hold them in your heart and soul, the more prepared you become to open to receive from the Entities.

With this process, you build, refine, and deepen the energy of your requests. You arrive at the Casa with focus, clarity, and preparation. Most likely, you'll be there for a short time, like two weeks. Even if you're there longer, you want to hit the ground running.

When you arrive at the Casa, you hold the energy of your requests in your body and field. This is what the Entities perceive. The paper on which you write your requests is unnecessary.

This process helps you do just that.

Hold these three requests as your main intentions for your journey.

What about my fifty-four other requests?

Make a long list of your fifty-four other requests (you don't need to prioritize them).

Soon after you arrive at the Casa, write your name, date of birth, and address on the list and put it in the triangle in the Great Hall or the other two triangles—whichever calls to you.

During the rest of your stay, feel free to make more requests each day. That way, even if you're not going before the Entity, you know your requests are being received. You also learn to ask for help from the higher realms on a regular basis.

All requests are seen by the Entities. All requests placed in the triangle are worked on for a year.

The mysterious part

You need to prepare your requests. Then you need to let go of them. That is, surrender.

This will happen at the Casa.

This is the mysterious part of surrender and trust. You need to boldly ask for what you want, but ask it within a light, spacious surrender, believing that the Entities know what you really need. Tricky, huh?

You get what you need, not what you want

After all your requests, you need to let go of them.

Huh? Yes.

You ask for what you want. And you may well get it. If so, wonderful!

But ultimately, you get what you need.

So, ask for the red convertible, but you may get a pink elephant, as you may be traveling in India in a dense forest with fairies, and this will suit you better. (Thanks to Catherine Tucker for this delightful insight.)

What you need may look very different from what you want or expect. It may be challenging, even outrageous. But the Entities and Spirit give you exactly what you need, whether directly or by a more circuitous route. Your spiritual or emotional lesson may be more important than getting what you want.

The best way to be with requests is to hold them as well as surrender to what is in your highest and best interest. Especially ones that you think you really, really need.

Many people get frustrated and think, "They're not helping me with this! I asked for this, but they gave me that!" There may be a lesson or gift in what they're giving you. You may have to learn or stretch or risk something first. There may be karma to be cleared. You may not be ready to receive what you want. Yet. It calls for patience. And growth. And learning to accept that this is what Spirit is delivering to you because it's what you most need.

Many say that what they receive is beyond what their logical mind could have imagined or asked for.

The magic is that you may receive something beyond, and more stupendous, than what you dare ask for.

Questions to
Ask Yourself . . .

"Have patience with everything
that remains unsolved in your heart.
Try to love the questions themselves, like locked rooms
and like books written in a foreign language."

—RAINER MARIA RILKE

Physical

IT'S HELPFUL TO list every physical issue you'd like help with. When you write it down, you bring it into your awareness. Writing things down makes your requests concrete to yourself, so you're more prepared.

- ◆ **Healing:** List everything for which you need healing. Diseases, conditions, aches, pains, old surgeries, even major wounds you had when you were little. Just write them down. You might be surprised by all that comes up. Your body holds your past, sometimes all too tightly. When you're aware of all you've dealt with, you're aware of and ready to heal. In this way, you help the Entities work on and with you.

◆ **Growth:** Ask the Entities to help you have the body you'd like to have. It might be to lose weight, or to help you get motivated to eat right or exercise. Remember, there's nothing too large or too trivial to ask for help with.

◆ Finally, reflect on what the emotional and spiritual connections to this issue might be.

Checklist:

List all the areas for which you want physical healing. They may be big or small. Recent or very old. With each one:

◆ What is the issue?

◆ When did it become an issue?

◆ How does it impact your life?

◆ What was happening in your life when it began?

◆ How do you imagine your life would look and feel if you didn't have it?

◆ What do you think, feel, or sense this is about for you? Emotionally? Spiritually?

◆ How do you eat?

◆ How do you exercise?

◆ What physically nourishes and nurtures you?

◆ How safe do you feel in the world?

◆ Do you have any self-limiting beliefs about your body? What are they?

◆ What would you like to have or manifest for yourself physically and materially?

◆ How do you feel physically on earth and this world?

  ◆ Do you feel like you belong?

  ◆ Do you feel safe and secure?

  ◆ Do you feel grounded?

  ◆ Do you feel supported?

◆ What is the health of your sexuality?

  ◆ Sexuality

  ◆ Sensuality

  ◆ Pleasure

  ◆ Desire

  ◆ Arousal

◆ Home

  ◆ What is home for you?

  ◆ Where is home for you? Where do feel at home?

- Imagine your perfect home. What does it look like?

- How does it compare with where you live now?

- What feels different between the two?

Emotional

Disease and illness are often manifestations of emotional wounding or trauma. Your body carries your life history in its bones, muscles, tissues, and cells.

Your emotional wounding or patterns may even carry over from past lives. The Entities help you clear and release your past-life karma, even if you don't know what that may be.

Things will come up at the Casa. Deep things. Old things. Things you think you've gotten over or healed. Even after you've done a lot of inner work, there are still deeper, unresolved layers.

Emotional healing with the Entities can
be a final processing and releasing of
old blueprints.

When you review and reflect on your emotional life, you prepare the ground for your emotional healing. Many of us don't tend to our emotional lives. But it's often the heart, the core engine, of your inner process. This process is like preparing the earth for sowing. It readies you to know what you may be working on and prepares you to dive into the deeper emotional current into which you're swept at the Casa. It helps you hit the ground running. It also helps you work with the Entities, for they will work as fast as you can go!

Just as your body carries its life history in its muscles and cells, it also holds the possibility for whole, vital, and strong emotional health, which includes love, joy, delight, courage, calm, and optimism. The Entities work with you to release negative emotions and live from positive ones.

Checklist:

◆ What is your emotional wounding?

◆ What traumas have you experienced?

◆ Of what are you afraid?

◆ What makes you angry?

◆ What makes you jealous?

◆ What or whom do you hate?

◆ What self-limiting beliefs do you hold as a result of your wounding or trauma?

◆ What do you shut out from yourself and your life? Or do you take in more than you can handle?

◆ What is the health of your power?

  ◆ How do you experience your personal power?

  ◆ Are you satisfied with how you feel and express your power?

  ◆ How do others experience your power?

- How do you respect and treat yourself? How don't you?

- What is the state of your self-esteem and confidence?

- How assertive are you?

- How aggressive are you?

- Are your relationships competitive or mutual? Are you satisfied with the power dynamics of your relationships?

◆ What is the health of your heart?

  - How and what do you love?

  - Are you satisfied by the ways that you love?

  - Is your heart open to yourself, others, and the world as you would like it to be?

  - In what ways do you not love? And would you like to love?

  - Do you receive enough love, care, friendship, tenderness, and emotional nourishment?

  - How do you receive love? Is it difficult to take in, or easy?

◆ How much of these positive emotions do you have in your life? Do you want more?

  - Joy

  - Possibility

- ◆ Delight

- ◆ Hope

- ◆ Fearlessness and courage

- ◆ Adventure

- ◆ Empathy

- ◆ Giving and receiving

- ◆ Awe and wonder

- ◆ Any other positive emotions

◆ If you could be the person you sense you might be without your wounding, who might you be? How would you feel? How would you act and move in the world?

Relationships

Relationships are the lifeblood of your emotional life. Family. Friends. Colleagues. Community. You are part of the network of life. As you heal, so do others. As you grow, so do others. Your healing is connected with others, and theirs with yours. You are interconnected; you live in connection and grow in healthy connection.

Relationships are the practice of love. They are love in practice, in process. Even and especially your most challenging relationships hold lessons and growth.

Relationships are also exchanges of energy. You may have taken on burdens placed on you when you were young that you need to return. Or you may have given parts of yourself, like your power, away to others, and you need to reclaim them. Relationship healing makes you more whole within yourself and with others.

The Entities heal you as well as
two generations before you. They
work on your lineage and heal
intergenerationally.

Think of every relationship that was and is important to you, whether the people are alive or have passed. If you find yourself thinking or dreaming of someone, they're significant! Especially bring in your most challenging or failed relationships, or those you've cut out for some painful reason. Just write them down, even if you don't know how to move forward with them. It's best if you don't have answers or ideas of how you'd like challenging relationships to change. Just be open to being with whatever feelings may come up around them.

How would you like your relationships to be?

Checklist:

◆ With each important relationship:

  ◆ What is the current state of this relationship?

  ◆ What is your emotional state with this person? Are you close or distant? Do you have positive or negative feelings toward them?

- ◆ How is this relationship helping you grow, even in ways that don't feel positive?

◆ Family

- ◆ Where are you now with this person?

- ◆ What have you received from this person?

- ◆ What have you not received?

- ◆ What have you given away?

- ◆ What is your deepest joy and pain?

- ◆ What are you grateful for?

◆ Difficult relationships

- ◆ Where are things now?

- ◆ What's at the heart of your feelings with them?

- ◆ In your wildest fantasy, how would you like this relationship to be?

◆ How much trust do you feel with others?

- ◆ How much mistrust?

- ◆ Have you been betrayed?

- ◆ How does your trust (or lack of trust) affect your current relationships?

- ◆ Who would you be if you could trust others?

- Work and professional community

  - What does your work or professional community look like?

  - Do you want to change or grow it in any way?

  - Are there ways in which you need support or mentoring?

  - Are there ways in which you would like to support or mentor?

  - Who would you like to be in the world?

  - What kind of community do you need to support you in your work?

- Personal community

  - What does your personal community look like?

  - Do you want to change or grow it in any way?

  - If so, in what ways?

  - What kind of community do you need and would you like to have?

- Friends

  - Do you have enough friends?

  - How do you feel about them?

  - Do you feel connected, supported, nourished, cared about, and loved?

- Do you have friends with whom to laugh and play and dance?

- Do you have friends who get you and your different aspects?

- Do you want to invite more and/or different kinds of friends into your life?

◆ How do you hold your power in relationships?

- How do you give to and receive from others?

- How independent or dependent are you?

- What is your power dynamic in relationships?

- What would you like more or less of?

◆ How open is your heart in relationships?

- How do you love?

- How do you turn away from love?

- How do you receive love?

Work, creativity, and life purpose

You may love your work. Or you may want to do something more meaningful.

Either way, there's room for more.

The Entities want you to develop your potential. They want to help you be successful. If you want to do something more meaningful, they can help you find your life purpose. They may help you access and bring forward talents you haven't used. If you're happy with what you do, they can help increase your capacity, competency, and creativity. They can help refine and expand your work.

Many report the Entities help them make professional connections and create opportunities beyond their expectations. Seeming synchronicities. Many feel the Entities guiding them in their decisions. And many are surprised to find a whole new line of work emerging after going to the Casa.

> The Entities help you manifest
> your soul potential and purpose.

Checklist:

- What is your deepest intention for your work?

- Does your work fully satisfy you?

- Are you aligned with what you do? Or do you feel or sense you could do something more? Something different?

- What do you fantasize about doing?

- Is there something you've longed to do but haven't?

- What in you longs to be expressed?

- Are there any talents you'd love to develop?

- How has your creativity been held back, not grown, or flourished?

◆ How would you like it to be renewed, nurtured, and nourished?

◆ If you could fully express your creativity, what would you create? Imagine how that might feel.

◆ In what ways does your personal power express or not get expressed in your work and creative life?

◆ Do you want to know your life purpose? If so, simply ask for the Entities' guidance when you go to the Casa.

◆ What is the health of your voice and creativity?

◆ What is your voice like to yourself? To others? In the world?

◆ Are you expressing everything you want to?

◆ What does your voice (self-expression) want to say? Speak? Sing? Shout? Draw? Build? Write? Create?

Energetic, psychic, and mediumship

Many people's intuitive, psychic, and mediumship capacities are validated, opened, and developed at the Casa.

Checklist:

◆ What are your gifts?

◆ What would you like to open to or develop?

- How intuitive are you? Would you like to develop your intuition more?

- Do you have any unexplained happenings or feelings?

- Do you have experiences that aren't validated by others?

- Does anything block you?

- Is anything happening that you'd like to clear?

- Are there energies around or within you that you'd like to clear but don't know how?

- Do you have psychic or mediumistic capacities or sensitivities? If so, would you like to develop them?

- If you're a sensitive, do you need to learn ways to protect yourself? Cleanse yourself?

- If you're a healer, what kinds of things do you want to learn to protect, cleanse, and heal for yourself and your clients?

- Would you like to develop your intuition? In what ways?

Money and material resources

If you struggle with money, this section is for you!

Money is so complex and complicated. It's tied into how you value yourself, what you think you deserve, and even what you allow yourself to have. It's connected to how supported and nourished you feel in the world. And it's often bound up with religious and spiritual beliefs, which often say you're not supposed to want money!

When I tell people I take to the Casa to ask for material resources, they're frequently shocked. Many are given and subscribe to the religious belief that spirituality and money are separate, that to really be spiritual, they should embrace scarcity and impoverishment.

Ah, but these are all "shoulds," aren't they?

Thinking that being spiritual implies being poor and dismissing money, the material world, or your body, is an imbalanced religious view, according to the Entities. They offer a very different take to that divided notion.

The Entities want you to live comfortably and well so you're not anxious and struggling. When you struggle, you become small, and attract what's constricted and limited.

If you're comfortable and have an easeful life, you live and create and share from inner spaciousness and generosity. The Entities want you to have abundance (whatever that looks like for you), so you can realize and manifest your full potential.

John of God himself is a successful and savvy businessman, even though he's illiterate. Having lived a life of hardship, he knows the value of having. He's set up soup kitchens for the poor and hungry, and helps many people grow their businesses in his regular life. The Entities have guided him with his business endeavors so he can provide for his family.

The Entities are extremely practical. They take great interest in your work since it's often connected to your life purpose. Since most of them have lived on earth, they understand your material needs.

Checklist:

- What is money for you?

- How do you feel about it?

- What is your relationship to money?

- What are your beliefs about money?

- Do your beliefs and feelings about money keep you small?

- In what ways do they connect with food, eating, and nourishment?

- How do you feel about others who have money?

- If you don't have enough:

  - Do you believe you can have it? Not have it? Shouldn't have it?

  - How deserving do you feel? How do you value yourself?

  - What do you want that would feel comfortable, supportive, and allow you to have the lifestyle you'd like to have? List the biggest and smallest things, even to the precision of a red convertible.

- If you have enough:

  - How do you use it?

  - Do you play and create with it?

- What kinds of things, events, and situations do you create from it? Do you feel good about these?

- Are you a steward for it?

- Do you share your abundance with others, either materially or by imparting your experience, knowledge, and expertise?

- How would you like to share? Give back? Pay it forward?

Growth

Here are some questions to mull over. You may have more.

Checklist:

- What do you want to call into your life?

- What do you want to manifest?

- Sit and connect with your heart and soul. What do you deeply long for?

- What calls or speaks to you? What has been calling you that you've been ignoring?

- Is there anything you hold yourself back from doing?

- What are some of your compelling dreams, intuitions, or fantasies?

- Do you feel or sense any repeated messages coming to you? These often may be in ways the rational mind doesn't understand, but in images, sensations, dreams, or knowings.

◆ Have you felt any misgivings about something that isn't quite right or can be different?

◆ Have you longed for something that seems outrageous and impossible, yet you keep returning to it even though you don't know how to get there?

◆ If you can imagine yourself without something you carry, who could you be? What would you do?

Spiritual

Would you like to open and connect more with the Divine or Spirit or God? In what ways?

How to Prepare Spiritually

"There is a candle in your heart, ready to be kindled.
There is a void in your soul, ready to be filled.
You feel it, don't you?"

—RUMI

Create space to do nothing

CREATE SPACE WHERE you can just be. Take a walk or hike in nature. Spread a blanket beneath a tree and lie down. Gaze at the sky. Take a trip to the beach or mountains if you're close, or to your favorite nature spot. Get away for a day or two, or even an hour or two.

If you're artistic and creative, engage in your favorite form of visual art, music, writing, dance or movement, or make a collage. Practice a craft like woodworking or knitting. Do whatever leads you to yourself, like cooking, gardening, watching a sunset, or just lying on your couch with nothing at all to do.

Do what gets you out of your mind, where you're connected with another way of knowing, sensing, intuiting.

When you create space, anything can happen. You make space for what isn't yet there to arrive. For what you don't yet know, for what is outside of what you know.

When you create space, you spread a blanket and invite possibility and potential.

Invite yourself

This is an opportunity to let everything else in your life drop away. It's all about you. Let go of family, work, friends, activities, the hustle and bustle of your life.

Invite your deepest self into this space.

Or set an intention to be fully present with yourself.

Observe your thoughts

Your mind needs to do its thing. It needs to stay busy, buzzing about your life. Allow it.

Notice what it keeps landing on or returning to. It could be a problem at work, a challenging relationship, or something else to which you are trying to find a solution. Anything. Whatever. If your mind keeps returning to it, just notice what it is. Make note of it.

Daydream

After your mind has raced all over your life, invite in your subconscious.

It's best to do this lying down.

Close your eyes. Breathe deeply a few times. Feel the full

length and width and breadth of your body, starting with your feet and going up to your head. Let your awareness slowly move from your toes, feeling into your muscles and tissues, bones, organs, and cells, all the way up to the crown of your head. Then move back down to your feet. Do this a few times.

Scan through your life as though it were a movie. Let whatever comes up float through you. They may be images, memories, or dreams you have had, peak moments or your most difficult, painful situations. What hopes and dreams haven't been realized? What do you know? And what have you felt at the edges or corners of your knowing, including the most strange, magical, wild, and out-of-this world?

Dream at night

Invite your subconscious at night. It loves to work at night. It's incredibly active, creative, and engages all that your conscious mind doesn't.

Before you sleep, invite your Higher Self, your soul, your highest purpose, your full potential, all that you are.

If you don't dream at night, ask to remember your dreamscape as you lie down to sleep. When you first wake up, don't jump right up, but allow yourself to remember. Whatever comes will be useful.

Invite your deepest intentions to come forward on your journey to John of God.

The subconscious speaks in images. So watch for images you may receive in the daytime. Even if you don't understand them, note them.

Tune in

Tune in to your heart. Tune in to your soul. Ask yourself:

- What do I want most deeply?

- What is my highest purpose?

- If I could be all that I can be, who would I be?

- What does that look like?

- How would I feel?

- Who have I dreamed of being? What have I dreamed of doing?

- If all the events and relationships that have hurt or held me back hadn't happened, who would I be?

On some fundamental level, you may have a sense of who you are, of all that you are. Be aware of those images, feelings, and knowings, however vivid or subtle. They might seem wild or crazy or ludicrous. Let yourself entertain them, even if only to entertain yourself!

Meditate

If you're a regular meditator, you know how to do this. You might consider making it more regular or devoting more time to it.

If you don't meditate, and the word meditation seems too lofty or spiritual, then try thinking of it as a time to connect with your deeper self. Or as a time to unplug and settle softly into your being.

Meditation is just being, not doing. Anyone can meditate. What's in the forefront of your experience right now? Is it pleasant or unpleasant? How are you responding to it? Watch for patterns like constantly diverting yourself when an unpleasant thought or sensation arises, or using force words like "I should" or "I must" stay open to this. In meditation we learn that we can be with our deepest experiences compassionately. And when your flow of thoughts and sensations slow down, just rest in that spaciousness.

Talk to your guides

Contact your guardian angel. Talk with your spirit guides. Talk to the Entities. If you haven't done this before, it can seem a little crazy. Talk to whom? But if you're planning on visiting John of God, you might want to get used to this. For the Entities are discarnate beings, as often your guardian angels and spirit guides are. If you don't believe in them, you might think of talking to the Universe or God or Goddess or Source or Spirit or . . . whatever you hold sacred.

Gratitude is a great way to make contact. When you express gratitude for something, however small, like the sunrise, your breakfast, or a warm hug, you raise your vibration, which makes it easier to connect.

You may try phrases like "dear guide," "Entities of Light and Love," "divine angels," "holy Ones," or "blessed beings." Or you might address whomever is sacred to you, like Jesus, Mother Mary, Buddha, Krishna, Shiva, Sophia, Allah . . .

Ask for their guidance. In everything. In preparing for your life. In preparing for your journey. Ask them to show you what you need to know, to see what you don't yet see, to be shown. And to understand clearly what their guidance is.

You can ask them to show you multiple times. Or ask for a sign. For guidance can be so subtle, it's easy to mistake it for your own fantasy and so disbelieve and disregard it.

Gratitude is a great way to end. Thank them for being with you, for their presence, grace, and blessings. Offer them what's in your heart.

How to Travel
with Others

"One must learn an inner solitude,
wherever one might be."

—Meister Eckhart

YOU MAY BE traveling with your spouse or partner, friend(s) or family. You may be a caretaker for a child, parent, or someone you're traveling with. It's wonderful to go with someone you know to share this experience. It's also good to be mindful of what you want for yourself and with each other.

There are pros and cons to traveling alone and to traveling with someone.

When you travel alone, you make all the decisions for yourself. You don't need to consult anyone. Your time, choices, and decisions are yours. You're open to what may happen. You're independent.

When you travel with someone, you get to share your

experiences. You don't need to seek out connection at the Casa. On the other hand, you need to balance your different needs: physical, emotional, spiritual, space, and togetherness. You may also be less open to other connections. You may or may not like having to consult and compromise with someone.

When you travel with someone, whether it's someone you know or in a group, it's a good exercise in growing. Your buttons can get pushed. Others serve as mirrors and reflections of you: what you see in them exists in you. And it's a great way to work on yourself, even with them if they're open to that.

My partner and I love traveling to the Casa together in a way that works for both of us. It gives us time to be with each other in a very special way. We stay at the same pousada in separate rooms and have lots of time apart, in solitude, and with other friends. We respect each other's space and connection with others. Every evening, often watching a glorious sunset, we share our day's process with each other. Knowing and having each other available when one of us is going through intense or profound experiences has been a beautiful, sacred way to deepen our relationship and spiritual connection.

We've also felt the Entities help us with whatever issue we've been working on in our relationship. Sometimes, we go before the Entity to get permission to go to the waterfall together. We've also gone before the Entity to ask for protection, blessings, and to make requests for ourselves as a couple.

Set an intention

Set an intention for your journey with each other. Some questions to ask yourself:

- What are you hoping for or expecting to achieve in traveling together?

- What is most important to you about traveling together?

- Is there something in your relationship you'd like to process while you're there?

- What do you think you want to give and receive from each other?

- In what ways do you want to support each other?

Balance relationships and solitude

Journeying to the Casa is like a retreat.

You may deeply value your solitude and personal process. Or you may love meeting others and hearing about their experiences and don't want to be alone. You may fall somewhere in between.

Your journey to the Casa is for you. You get to dive into your process deeply when you spend a lot of time meditating and reflecting. While it's great to share what feels right with someone, be discerning as to how much, what, and when. Find a balance between solitude and connection that helps you focus on your process.

Honor your process. Are you the kind of person who gives up what you need for others? Are you the kind of person who will find connection so you don't have to be alone?

- How much time do you want to spend together and alone?

- What do you want for yourselves individually and with each other?

- What kinds of boundaries would you like?

Solitude

Solitude helps you maintain your focus on your inner process, which is so essential for your healing journey. It may or may not be easy for you. If it's uncomfortable or difficult, you might explore why.

It's good to connect and share with people and make new friends, but watch out for socializing becoming a distraction from your inner process. Remember, you're on a spiritual retreat, where you have much to gain in quiet contemplation, reflection, and meditation.

Should we share a room?

- Unless you're going with small children, I recommend you not share a room. One or both of you are likely to have surgery, for which it's very important to have your personal space. Surgery opens your spiritual aura and you don't want anybody else's energy in there, no matter how close you are. Surgery is your individual process, not a couple's process. If one of you has surgery and the other doesn't, you'll have very disparate experiences. Couples who've shared rooms discover that the person having surgery finds the other's presence intrusive. And the one who hasn't had surgery wants to give his or her partner space, which means finding a place to hang out other than the room. Not ideal!

Surgery frequently brings on physical releases like headaches, diarrhea, and vomiting. One bathroom can feel much too small! Also, many feelings and emotions arise, some of which could be about the person you're with. It's really important to have your personal space in which to fully experience your personal process.

◆ Keep boundaries in mind. Do you really want to share everything with your partner, parent, or friend? It's a great time to take personal space.

◆ If you're a caretaker for someone, you'll receive lots of your own healing. The Entities support you both. It's a time for you to rest and receive as well.

Samantha, Bob's wife, has been his sole caretaker for the past eight years as a result of his cancer. He hasn't been able to do much for himself, and she came to the Casa weary, depleted, and worried. Both of them had multiple surgeries, and Samantha was surprised by the time she had to herself and the depths of grief over the loss of her relationship and life as a result of Bob's cancer. Letting go of taking care of him and feeling the Entities supporting both of them helped her face and process some of how she takes responsibility for others at the cost of herself.

◆ Most pousadas charge by person, not by room. Two people sharing a room is almost the same cost as individual rooms. So there's no savings when you room together.

Logistics

"I am glad you are here with me.
Here at the end of all things, Sam."

—J.R.R. TOLKIEN

Do I need a guide?

I HIGHLY RECOMMEND THAT you go with a guide the first time you visit the Casa.

It's radically different from visiting a foreign country. The paradigm of the Casa is completely different from anywhere you've been.

Some reasons to hire a guide:

◆ A guide takes care of logistics and helps you with decisions at every choice point. You don't have to figure everything out.

◆ When you hire a guide, you can focus on your inner process and not worry about navigating this totally new environment. You give yourself an opportunity to fully drop into your inner process and leave the logistics to someone else (so helpful when traveling beyond the veil!).

◆ The numerous Casa protocols and possibilities are bewildering to first-time visitors. It's easy not to follow all the protocols and miss some. But all details prescribed by the Entities are important for your healing. When you hire a guide, you don't have to know it all—they shepherd you through each step, reminding you of everything you need to remember.

◆ When you don't know anyone in a sea of people, it's great to have your guide to talk with and share your experiences.

I highly recommend using an authorized Casa guide, especially on your first trip.

Visit www.abadianiaportal.com or www.friendsofthecasa. info for guide listings. You can hire a guide exclusively for yourself or go with a group.

Guides' fees are set by the Casa and usually include your room, board, and travel to and from Brasilia. Each guide's offerings vary slightly, but they're all within a close range. You pay a little more than if you were going on your own, but you receive substantial value in return.

Brazil: A new culture

If you're not Brazilian and haven't visited Brazil, you're entering a new culture.

Brazilians are a very friendly, open, warm, and animated people. They do things differently, with much more fluidity and accommodation of multiple perspectives. They may have a different approach to time than yours. It is easy, given the number of American and European visitors, to expect Abadiania and the Casa to function in a way and with perspectives familiar to you.

Yet you are a visitor in Brazil, where customs are different and may sometimes even seem strange. Honor and respect these differences, and if you don't understand something, ask a local to explain a custom or manner. Bear in mind that you may not know the context or reason for how things are organized or done, particularly at the Casa. You may naturally impose your expectations, have judgments, and project onto people, the environment, or the situation. Be aware of them. Like everything else, while visiting there, chances are that whatever comes up for you is fodder for your inner work.

The best way to navigate the culture is to enjoy, appreciate, and be open to different perspectives and ways of relating and living. Visiting Abadiania might challenge aspects of yourself or your life. The best way is to go with the flow.

Resources for travel

- www.friendsofthecasa.info
- www.abadianiaportal.com

What Happens at the Casa?

"And suddenly you know: It's time to start something new and trust the magic of beginnings."

——MEISTER ECKHART

WHEN YOU ARRIVE in Abadiania, a team of Entities begins working with you. They know what you need and work with you for your entire stay. Going before the Entity is not the only time you're "seen" or treated; you're worked on 24/7 by your very own personal team of Spirit doctors.

At the Casa

You may feel the powerful energy as you enter the Casa gates. Intensive healing happens in Abadiania and at the Casa no matter what you're doing, and not just while you're before the Entity. Whether you're strolling through the garden, sitting on a meditation bench, standing in line for soup, or waiting in the Great Hall, every moment is an opportunity to receive.

Tune in to your experience. Open to receiving. Among the chatting crowds, it's easy to treat waiting in line as a social event, like a movie or show, but so much happens all the time. You're being prepared and worked on by teams of Entities every moment.

What's the difference between "Entities" and "the Entity"?

The term "the Entities" is used to refer to the group, the phalange of beings in Abadiania and the Casa that work on people.

"The Entity" is a single being working through John of God during a Casa session. John of God channels multiple entities, but only one is incorporated in Medium João's body at any moment in time. When incorporated, John of God is referred to as "the Entity." When John of God is not in session, he is referred to as Medium João.

Going before the Entity

You can go before the Entity once a day, unless you've been invited for surgery, the two o'clock line, or if the Entity has asked you to come again. Before you go in line your first time, get your three requests translated by the Casa translators or your guide.

When you go before the Entity, you're asking for help. Your requests are your participation in your healing. When you make requests, you give the Entities permission to work on you. The Entities read your entire blueprint: your past, present, and future possibilities. Along with your requests, ask to know, release, or shift what you need to so that you become more aligned with yourself, heal, and open to your gifts. These would be things you don't know, so you can't ask about them. This is the first step.

The second step is, while you wait in the Great Hall and as you walk in line and stand before the Entity, to open up, let go, surrender, and trust as much as you are able that whatever you receive from the Entities and the Divine is in your highest and best interest. The Entities know what you need. And healing can be in an order unknown to you. For instance, you may need to shift X, R, and G before healing Z.

Words are unnecessary when you go before the Entity. Everything about you is known. Your requests are an exercise for you, your own inner preparation, not necessarily words and sentences that you need to make sure are correctly communicated and translated. Likewise, the Entity doesn't explain your healing process to you because it is too complex, of a different paradigm, and might only create worry and confusion. They focus on healing you, not telling you about the process or what you're healing from. But you might and often will know because of your feelings, thoughts, memories, and dreams.

As you approach the Entity, be sure to make eye contact with and hand your requests to a translator. When you're right before the Entity, look into his eyes if he looks at you. Often, he will have his left palm outstretched or extend it toward you. Place your right hand on it. Sometimes, you may experience a wave or transmission of energy. These are powerful ways you connect with the Entity.

Usually your time before the Entity is very brief. You might hear your treatment before the translator finishes (or begins!) reading your requests. You may wonder whether everything was known, but be assured that, regardless of how brief your interaction, the Entity knows everything about you and you're being worked on.

When the Entity looks at the person behind you, or the translator tells you what was communicated, please move on. Make sure you understand all communication from the translator before leaving. If you don't understand it, ask the translator to repeat it. With hundreds passing before the Entity, translators cannot remember individual messages later.

Subsequent times

Once you've made a request, you don't need to keep making it. Going in line again and again isn't really necessary, especially since the Entities know what you need even before you get there. Making the same request multiple times doesn't make the Entities work any faster. Remember, you're receiving everything you need and in the order you need it. Open. Trust. Surrender. Let go. If you haven't received healing or an answer, know that the Entities are working on it. You may want to sit with why you haven't received it for guidance and healing in Current or in meditation.

Josie RavenWing, a long-time, experienced Casa guide, has had several discussions with the Entity Dr. Augusto, who said, "It's actually better for people to pass by just once a week, then spend the rest of the time (unless they're having surgery or resting from it) going to Current if they're able to, because so much work happens there."

Bob Dinga and Diana Rose, long-time guides, tell the story of a woman who put her long list of requests in the triangle on a Wednesday. The next day, she went before the Entity with her short list of three requests. Worried that the Entities needed to know everything, she asked the translator to also read her long list, a copy of the one she had put in the triangle. As soon as the translator began, the Entity said, "We just got this list on Wednesday. It's only been one day! We're working on it."

After your first time, tune in to yourself before you go in line each time—you'll have gone through a process since your previous time. New things may come up that you want to request. Or you may want to make one of the many other requests on your list. Remember, you can make up to three requests. Trust your intuition and guidance. The Entity will give you whatever treatment you need at this point in time in order to advance to your next level.

You can also choose voluntary surgery if it is offered and you feel so guided. You don't need the Entity's permission if you've gone before him at least once each visit.

Translation

There are helpful volunteer translators available at the Casa who translate your requests into Portuguese. They will quickly word, interpret, and condense your requests into a few words. If you have a long or complicated request, they'll intuitively help shape it for you. There is also a cultural translation. For instance, a request for spiritual growth is often worded as "mediumship."

Many are often disappointed when their long requests get translated into one or a few words. Know that you hold your requests within you. And all your information is always accessible to the Entities. So when you go before the Entity, you may be waved along even before your requests are read. This is because everything about you is already known.

They know your requests from your energy field. By what you hold in your body, your heart, your soul. They don't require words on a piece of paper. Then again, sometimes the Entity may ask you questions or talk to you about your requests. Above all, know that they're working intimately with you, regardless of how your requests are worded.

Let go. Open. And receive.

Crystal bed

The crystal bed is a wonderful treatment through which the Entities work on you.

When you arrive at the Casa, crystal bed sessions are a great way to begin your healing and raise your vibration before the Casa days begin. You can sign up for crystal bed sessions at the bookstore; you don't need the Entity's permission. Sessions are in twenty-minute segments, and you can have up to an hour's treatment every day.

Prepare an intention before you have a session. It's good to go ten to fifteen minutes before your session and sit on the benches or in the waiting area. Hold your intention as you prepare to open to and receive your healing.

During the session, you don't have to "do" anything. Just lie there. Everything and anything that needs to come up will come up. Just be with it. Feel it. You will be guided and shown what you need. All you have to do is receive.

Some people feel physical symptoms like heat, tingling,

energy currents, or even discomfort. You may feel deeply relaxed and even sleep. If you do, it is exactly what you need, for much of your healing happens when you are deeply resting. You may have old or past-life memories with their accompanying emotions arise. You may shift your perspective on a situation or your life. You may experience beings or loved ones who've passed. You may receive messages and guidance. You may have amazing spiritual experiences.

Whatever your experience, however clear or obscure, it's important to know that you've received exactly what you need. Some feel deeply; some may experience very little or nothing at all. Just be open to all that you experience.

After your session, spend some time on the benches or in the Casa garden to integrate and digest what you've received.

Current

Current is one of the most powerful healing experiences at the Casa. There are thousands of Entities working on you while you sit in Current. You are worked on directly and individually by the Entities. Many people have been healed during Current. A lot gets lifted out from you, and your energy becomes more equalized, aligned, and balanced.

Dr. Augusto directly told Josie RavenWing, a Casa guide, "We (the Entities) wish people would spend more time in Current (rather than in line) so that we can actually GIVE them what they're asking for!"

Current is also a unique way to give back and serve while receiving your own healing. Your body, or ectoplasm, is used by the Entities to generate and sustain the healing energy field while they work on you and others. When you sit in Current, you support the Entities' work. Service is a beautiful way to evolve, as the Entities do. It's good karma.

It is best to approach Current with your intentions and an open willingness to be with and look at yourself and your situations. Reflect on your intentions before you sit in Current. Ask from your open heart to be shown, guided, and helped. Or just ask to be shown whatever you need to be shown.

People receive all kinds of guidance. You may be shown how to work with different situations and experiences, like relationships, money, career, psychic and energy bodies, and your illness, if any. You may understand the cause of a situation from a spiritual perspective. You may process emotionally. You may see images, hear instructions or guidance, or just know a truth. You may feel sensations or discomfort. Your spiritual nature may be revealed, and you may travel to different dimensions. You may see visions of light, experience beings working with or on you, have conversations with them, and feel an incredible, exalted love. You may experience the profound sacredness of who you are and your existence in a way you never have before.

It's helpful to take a cushion with you to sit on during Current. The benches have foam padding, but their backs are wooden. Current can be as long as five hours or more, so if you have a bad back, or just want to be comfortable for long sittings, pack a cushion or a pillow. The pousadas do not like you taking their pillows to the Casa, so pack your own.

Sacred waterfall

The waterfall, or *cachoeira* in Portuguese, is a sacred, magical place. It is a very powerful energy stream full with the presence of Entities, devas, and nature spirits. You will receive much healing, guidance, and many blessings here.

You need the Entity's permission to go to the waterfall.

Please read and be mindful of the rules on signs en route and just before you enter the area. It is your way to offer your respect for the peace and sacredness of this healing body.

Say a prayer before entering. You may have an intention or want to open to whatever you receive. Stay open to messages while going to and under the waterfall, which may come as images, knowings, or voices you hear in your inner (or outer) mind.

Please observe silence as you wait your turn. Often there are long lines; please be mindful of others and not linger beyond your allotted time. It helps the flow to dress quickly. You don't need to dry off, since the water is healing as it dries on you. To be mindful of others in line, wear minimal clothing, like a cover-up, to reduce your time changing clothes.

You may be delightfully surprised by brilliant butterflies that rest on your body at the waterfall. Butterflies are often manifestations of the Entities at the Casa and at the waterfall in particular. Healing visitations and blessings, and sometimes butterflies, will stay on you for a while.

Triangle

The triangle in the Great Hall is a powerful portal. You can find photographs online that capture spirit energy flowing from it to people. You may experience it as very powerful. There have been remarkable healings and miracles from the triangle.

People stand before the triangle to pray and make requests. You will see people place their palms on the arms of the triangle while resting their head against the wall.

You can put family's and friends' pictures and requests in it for Entities' blessings. If someone asks you to put their picture in the triangle, get their picture with their name, date of birth, address including country, and requests, and place it there. You can make as many requests as you wish, unlike the limit of three when you go before the Entity.

You can also ask for a blessing for someone without needing their permission. Except you can't write your requests *for* them, only their contact information and date of birth. If you don't have a picture, you can just write their information on a piece of paper and place it there.

You don't need to put *your* picture in it because you're physically there!

There are two more triangles at the Casa: one is King Solomon's triangle, behind the healing rooms; the other is in an alcove in the Casa gardens. Use whichever one calls to you.

Blessed water

Drinking blessed water is an integral part of healing at the Casa. The water is blessed by the Entities, and it is recommended that you drink one to two liters a day. It flushes out physical, emotional, energetic, and other toxicities and brings Light into your body and field. When possible, drink from a cup so the source bottle doesn't get contaminated by bacteria from your mouth.

Casa protocols and orientation

Consult the *Official Casa Guide* for a detailed, precise layout of the Casa, the various lines, and a description of Casa protocols.

If you're a first-time visitor, I *strongly* recommend the Tuesday evening orientation at the Casa. The protocols change from time to time, so if you're visiting again, you also might want to attend the Casa orientation on Tuesday evening to get updated.

How to Process in Abadiania

"Perhaps all the dragons in our lives are princesses who are only waiting to see us act, just once, with beauty and courage. Perhaps everything that frightens us is, in its deepest essence, something helpless that wants our love."

—RAINER MARIA RILKE

Working with what comes up

EMOTIONS WILL COME up. They may be deep and intense. They may be overwhelming or subtle, fleeting or lasting, dark or light. They are all essential for your healing.

My experience of healing at the Casa is that it's like therapy at the speed of light with unconditional Love. When you open, you're guided to precisely what you need to process.

When you feel difficult feelings like grief, pain, hurt, loss, disappointment, anger, hate, and jealousy, simply be with them.

You may cry a lot. Physically, you may feel nauseous, vomit, be exhausted, or have headaches, diarrhea, skin outbursts, or rashes. Your symptoms may intensify, as in a Herxheimer or detox reaction, and you may feel worse. *This is all part of the healing.* Things are brought up in order to be lifted out of your body and energy field.

You don't have to do anything—often, you can't. Just open to each feeling and its nuance. When you feel your emotions fully, they get lifted out of you, out of your cells and body, out of your emotional, psychic, and energy fields. Out of your aura.

"Up and out" is how Barbara Rose Billings, a Daughter of the Casa and guide, describes working with emotions at the Casa. "You feel them, then they come out of you."

If it gets very intense, ask the Entities to help you in your process. Ask to be shown what you need to know.

What you need to learn is often outside of what you know. The path to your lesson and healing is through your feelings. The process leads you there. The Entities lead you there. All you need to do is fully participate by feeling, being with what's present, and staying open to what you don't yet know.

If you find yourself fiercely holding on to an issue which keeps coming up, chances are that you need to shift it. Sometimes, you may not even know what needs to shift. Once, I was absolute and rigid about a situation. I had a terrible headache for several days. Now I know a particular kind of headache is the way the Entities work on me. Initially, I struggled and resisted, since I was so invested in the outcome I wanted. When the headache became debilitating, I finally surrendered and asked to be shown what I didn't want to see. Within a few moments, I knew what shifts I needed to make and my headaches stopped then and there.

So ask the Entities for help, and keep asking them.

Opening to and going with the flow

Your process at the Casa is like stepping into a river. It's a flow, like a river, that carries you. It also contains discrete choice points, or drops of water.

Each moment is an opportunity—everything you need is available to you. You participate in each moment with your presence and the quality of your presence.

Each moment, each hour, each day is different. You will need something different today than what you needed yesterday. Tune in to what you need and be present with what is.

Solitude and socializing

Going to the Casa is to be on retreat. It's a time to go inside yourself, reflect, rest, and receive as much healing as you can take away. It's a time to be with yourself.

- **Solitude enhances what you receive.** Whether you're in the Great Hall, on the meditation benches, or resting in your pousada, solitude is a main part of your healing work.

- **Take time for solitude.** Tune in to your experience. Open to receiving. Moment by moment, hour by hour, ask yourself, "What do I need now?" It's a great way to be with what's important.

- **Take care of yourself.** You'll find yourself wiped out, sick, processing intense emotions, or just wanting to be alone. Honor your experience—this is your healing time. Protect and safeguard it. If you're not feeling social, honor that and take a tray to your room, sit apart from the group at a table by yourself, or just let people know when they approach you that you want to be alone. They will honor and respect your experience.

- **Minimize socializing.** There's a difference between socializing and communing. Socializing so you don't have to be alone with yourself or whiling away the time can distract you from your healing time and experience. Remember, you're primarily there for yourself.

- **Silence.** If you want to maintain silence for a few hours, a day, or several days while at the Casa, let people around you know and wear a sign.

- **Be discerning and mindful about whom you spend time with, how much time you spend, and what you share with whom.** If you feel too pulled out of your process, ask yourself whether you're socializing too much or with the right people. There are all kinds of people who visit the Casa, and you may need to set boundaries. If you feel like you're talking about things in which you have no interest, there's no need to stay to be polite. It's not a party or social occasion at which you're expected to chit chat and make small talk. Appreciate and acknowledge the other person's presence and time, then let him or her know you want to be alone to meditate, or go to your room.

- **Socialize at mealtimes.** At your pousada, mealtimes are a great time to share experiences and learn about the Entities, John of God, and the miracles happening around you. It's especially illuminating to talk with guides or people who've been there a few times.

- **Significant relationships.** Many people meet and make meaningful and significant connections at the Casa. You will know when that happens because you will feel a connection with that person or persons. These are good connections to nurture even after you return home, if you so choose.

Consideration of others

Everyone is at the Casa for their own deep healing process. When you want to share, be mindful of the other person. Be considerate of whether they're in their own process or in an emotional wave. Do they want your company or want to be alone? Can they be present with and hold what you want to share with them? One good way to know is to ask them explicitly whether they want company or want to be alone.

How to Prepare for Re-entry and Your Post-Casa Transition

"What you seek is seeking you."

—Rumi

How to protect your energy during return travel

BEFORE YOU LEAVE Abadiania, spend some time preparing for your return. For days, you've been in a protected, safe bubble of the Entities' energy and adjusted to its high frequency. Leaving this bubble can be jarring.

Ask the Entities for protection during your return travel. Ask at the triangle, in Current, or while meditating. You may receive guidance on how to protect yourself. One way to protect yourself energetically is to visualize a bubble around you through which no negative energy can enter, like white light of the highest frequency, a color, or roses.

Check and double-check your taxi and flight reservations. If you've signed up for alerts, make sure everything's in order. It's best to leave Abadiania four to five hours before your flight, depending on traffic.

As you drive out from Abadiania you might notice the shift in energy as you get on the freeway and, most likely, as you enter Brasilia. The crowds and lines at the airport can feel overstimulating. Keep visualizing your bubble.

No heavy lifting is one of the post-surgery guidelines. If you're within the forty days after surgery, it's very important not to lift your suitcase during any portion of the journey. It's even more important if you haven't had revision (a post-surgery procedure) after your most recent surgery, since you have stitches. When you get out of the taxi, ask your taxi driver to place your suitcase on one of the nearby luggage carts so you don't have to lift it.

The Brazilian airline customer service representatives are very friendly and helpful. They're very familiar with people returning from John of God, so do ask for extra assistance in lifting your suitcase onto the scale.

En route, don't be shy about asking for assistance if your carry-on bag is heavy and you need help lifting it into the overhead bins. People are often very willing to help with such matters. If you're hesitant, you can say that you've had surgery. It's true!

At customs in your arrival country, ask someone to help you lift your suitcase off the conveyer belt onto a cart. Ask whoever is picking you up to carry it into your home so you can unpack it without strain.

Getting the most from your healing

Stay connected with the Entities

You're connected with the Entities now; keep your inner conversation and communication with them going when you need or want anything, whether it's guidance, clarity, healing, or their presence.

Participate!

Your participation in your healing and growth continues after you return home. Just as when you were at the Casa, your participation is fifty percent of your process, and the Entities do the other fifty percent. Following the protocols is an essential way in which you participate. Consult the *Official Casa Guide* for all the protocols.

Create time and space for solitude

The number one thing I suggest to people who travel with me is, "create as much space and time for yourself as possible after you return." You will probably notice how different you feel because you've been in a high vibrational field so different from your regular world. You may feel emotionally or energetically raw, delicate, or fragile.

You may feel overwhelmed by what was normal for you before you went to the Casa. You may be jarred by the difference in your energy as compared to others'. You may discover that you feel and process things very differently.

This is good—it shows how much you've shifted and that you're tuned in to your healing process. Your challenge is protecting yourself from the waves of different energies that bombard you after your return.

So carve out as much space for solitude as possible. If you don't have to work or spend much time working, you can devote chunks of time to your healing process. If you have a job, reserve your mornings, evenings, and weekends for yourself. If you're a parent, create periods for solitude in your day. Ask your partner, family, and friends for their support.

Some people feel a natural shift around the forty-day mark after surgery. Others take months to a year to adjust.

Engage in healing activities in healing environments

The Entities work with you on obvious as well as incredibly subtle levels at the Casa and continue to do so after your return. You also continue to participate. Feelings, physical sensations, insights, perceptions, and guidance will continue to come to you as your process unfolds. Tune in to your process to support and flow with the healing waves coming toward you.

- ◆ Meditative and physical activities like yoga or tai chi that keep you connected with yourself.

- ◆ Nature is a wonderful environment that supports your vibration and process.

- ◆ Artistic activities like writing, music, visual arts, or movement are lovely ways to keep your process unfolding.

- ◆ Simple, creative activities like cooking, gardening, woodworking, sewing, or knitting are ways to be "doing something" while also being with yourself.

◆ Journaling is a great way to record your process. Or you may just choose to glide down the river of your becoming without needing to write.

Minimize external stimulation

Another way to protect your healing process is not to engage in anything overstimulating, jarring, and draining. When you protect what you've received, you increase and maximize your healing.

Socializing, shopping, TV, entertainment, and the trivial, mundane things in life are some ways in which you can drain and lose some of the energy you've received. We'll talk about dealing with people a little later in this chapter.

Hopefully, you've organized your life so that you're not going to shopping malls or have big purchases to make after you return. Similarly, avoid too much TV, loud music, horror movies, and anything that's out of sync with the Entities' energy.

Think gentle, soothing, soft, nourishing, playful, spacious.

Follow Casa protocols

This is extremely important. Remember, for forty days after your first surgery at the Casa, the protocols are to abstain from:

◆ sex, sexual activity, and any rise in sexual energy. This means not getting aroused, excited, or stimulated. This is a hard one! When you start feeling sexual energy, distract yourself: do something else, go for a walk, or call a friend. This energy has such a different vibration than the Entities' that they find it difficult to work while it's moving in your body. There are stories of people who were sexual during their forty days and their healing stopped or reverted until the next time they visited the Casa.

◆ no alcohol or drugs

◆ no heavy lifting or exercise for eight days after your last surgery.

◆ don't receive energy healing for forty days. Don't give it for eight days after your last surgery.

Bob Dinga, long-time Casa guide, was almost blind when he first visited the Casa for a day and a half. Not quite believing or understanding the severity of his surgery, he toured the countryside and shopped for crystals in the twenty-four-hour post-surgery period. By the end of the day, he was exhausted and his eyesight began to get worse. When he arrived back home, his ability to read diminished to almost zero without strong magnification, and he couldn't drive. He received guidance that he needed to visit the Casa two more times, after which his eyesight improved significantly. Now he leads a normal life.

Tune in

You're undergoing a profound transformation and birthing a new you. Stay tuned in to your experience, feelings, insights, and dreams so you're aware of and work with all that's shifting.

If you're in pain or discomfort, keep asking the Entities for healing and support. You might also ask to know the cause of what you're experiencing and for help to release it.

What to focus on

There's an overarching lesson or something uniquely important for you to learn and open to. That is why you were called to the Casa. That process has opened up. Stay open to what the lesson and growth might be for you. Keep asking yourself:

- ◆ What is all this about for me?

- ◆ What is it I don't yet know?

- ◆ What is it I need to change in myself? In my life?

In the weeks and months, even years, after you return from the Casa, you'll find yourself discovering more and more why you originally went, which may not seem connected to your original intention. Yet, in some way, it is.

You may realize that what you went there for was a gift, a blessing.

How to Stay Connected to the Entities

"That which God said to the rose,
and caused it to laugh in full-blown beauty,
He said to my heart,
and made it a hundred more times beautiful."

—RUMI

Meditation

MEDITATING EVERY DAY is one of the best ways to stay connected.

Crystals

If you bought crystals at the Casa store or had a crystal blessed by the Entity or while sitting in Current, hold it while you meditate, sit, or lie in bed to create a strong connection with the Entities. Holding it on or against a part of your body that's in pain or discomfort, or needs healing or support, can be very powerful.

Having crystals in your home, especially where you frequently sit or beside your bed, keeps you connected to the energy. Some crystals may be too powerful to have just beside your bed; experiment with where you want them in your bedroom.

If you hold crystals while you meditate or against your body, it's good to cleanse and clear them every three weeks or so. Soak them in sea salt for twenty-four hours or keep them in direct sunlight or moonlight.

Herbs

Herbs are a direct, ongoing way to stay connected since they are prescribed uniquely for you. They're like mini-visits before the Entity. Take them mindfully to participate in your healing and growth.

Hold your intention in your heart as you take them: these can be the intentions you made when you visited, had a distance healing, or whatever you need this moment. And it's always great to offer gratitude to the Entities.

If you finish your herbs and found them helpful, consider asking for a distance healing from someone who's visiting there, or by finding a guide online.

Rosary

If you bought a rosary from the Casa store, saying it or holding the beads in your palm keeps you connected.

Visualization

Visualize yourself at the Casa, in the healing rooms, in front of the Entity, by the outlook, at the triangle, or in any place that felt particularly powerful during your visit. It's a great way to stay connected.

Drink blessed water

You can carry back some blessed water bottles from the Casa in your suitcase. And drink a few drops or add them to a glass of water.

You can also make your own blessed water at home. Combine Casa water and regular water in the proportion of 1:2 into a container. For example, the one-liter Casa bottles fill a third of a gallon jar. Fill the remaining two-thirds with regular water. Let it sit for twenty-four hours (you can stick affirmations on it if you like!), and the entire gallon becomes blessed water. You can then keep making batches of blessed water, just as you would a yeast, yogurt, or kombucha starter. Make sure to thoroughly wash the jars every two to three weeks to avoid bacterial contamination.

Note: You will likely hear varying versions of the correct proportions; this isn't a baking recipe, but more of a general guideline.

Sit in Current

If your time zone allows, sit in Current when Casa is in session, Wednesday through Friday (Brazil time).

If you know other people near you who've been to John

of God, you can get together for a meditation or a "Current sitting" on a regular basis.

Triangle

If you bought a triangle, you can use it as a portal just like the ones at the Casa. Stand before it and place your forehead in the middle of it and pray, make your requests, or simply connect. It can be very powerful.

Casa music and pictures

Stay connected by playing CDs you bought at the Casa store or putting up pictures of John of God, the Entities, and even the little pamphlet you receive after you go before the Entity. All these bring Casa energy into your home.

Make your own rituals

Come up with your own rituals. Also, you may have received guidance while there about how to stay connected.

Crystal bed

If you are fortunate enough to have brought back a crystal bed or live close to someone who has one, regular sessions are a powerful way to continue your healing work. Crystal beds are a portal to the Entities and Casa. People have amazing experiences and healing with them.

Try to wear light colors for a crystal bed session, although it's not mandatory. Meditate and hold your intentions before each session, just as you would at the Casa, and sit for a while afterward to hold and deeply receive.

The crystal bed offers numerous uses and treatments. Michael Quinn in Pennsylvania uses it to assist the terminally ill with their transition.

Cultivate community

Keeping in touch with friends you made while in Abadiania is a lovely social way to stay connected and build community. Sharing your experiences with those who've visited the Casa raises your vibration and validates your experiences, since it can be hard to share them with those who haven't been there.

Join Friends of the Casa newsletter and Facebook

Sign up to receive the Friends of the Casa newsletter. It's great for receiving news, healing stories, and staying connected.

If you're on Facebook, they also have a Facebook page.

Books and DVDs

Reading books and watching DVDs you bought about John of God and Spiritism are other ways to stay connected. You may discover that your taste in movies changes after you return: after most visits, I can only watch spiritual movies and have discovered several Catholic movies on Netflix! Refer to the resources section for some book and film suggestions.

What can I expect?

Your healing process after being at the Casa is only a beginning.

Many people continue to have intense physical or emotional processes. You may feel like you're getting worse physically.

You may have difficult, intense days, but these are all part of the healing process. And remember, the Entities heal you on a spiritual level, and it takes a while for the healing to percolate outward through your energy, emotional, mental, and physical bodies. Think of it as a spiritual Herxheimer reaction. When it's getting worse, you're really getting better because you're releasing.

If and when it gets really bad, keep asking the Entities for their help. Ask them to ease your pain and discomfort. Ask them to show you what the issue is. Ask them to guide you to resources and people who can help you. Often, when you become conscious of the issue, the Entities clear it. Pain, discomfort, and unease are all mechanisms through which they help you get to the actual issue, which may feel like it's not related to your physical symptoms.

For instance, when I get a particular kind of headache that lasts for days, I know the Entities are working on something I'm particularly dense about or don't want to look at. It shifts when I finally surrender by asking them for their help to see or change what I'm so defended against.

You might release through your skin. You may get acne or skin disorders. Your digestion and elimination may be thrown off.

You may discover that your body feels different. Many report sleeping or eating less (or more), and that their cellular makeup feels different, new.

Emotionally, you might find yourself crying a lot, feeling emotions you haven't felt before, or things arising from the past. Your dreams may be vivid. You may receive guidance and messages.

Your perspectives and feelings toward relationships and situations may shift. What was charged may change and you may find you have more emotional capacity.

What you consider "weird" may happen. Pay attention to these experiences. Write them down even if you don't believe them, trust them, or know what to do with them. It's very possible that a new dimension of yourself has opened and is receiving information, guidance, and healing that your mind doesn't know what to do with. I often write these down, only to discover what they mean for me months or years later.

You may have made a huge shift. When your vibration changes, your world changes as well. You may no longer resonate with and may let go of activities, situations, and things you once connected with. Relationships may drop away. You might find yourself longing for new friends with whom you can connect and share your energy, experience, and vibration. New people may enter your life. You might be interested in new activities.

You might experience big and small miracles.

You might reevaluate many things or everything about you and your life!

You might question what you do, and discover your new purpose, work, and environments.

You might move to a new place.

You might find resources and opportunities manifesting.

All this shows your transformation!

Dealing with people

After going home can [?]

Your friends and family will be curious. You may be bursting to tell others about what you've experienced. You might experience others wanting more of you and your time.

Don't tell them.

Why not? Because the energy you've received and are holding is so powerful, subtle, and unique to you that people will usually notice it. They will sense something different about you, even though they won't have words for it. Many will be curious about your experience from their reality and want to know "whether you've healed." It's one thing to share with people who've been to the Casa or understand your spiritual process. It's another to speak about your experience to answer people's questions, even if they care.

Part of how you continue to keep the energy with you is by not revealing details of your healing process. Subtly working and unfolding in you, it takes weeks and months to integrate. The time to share with others is after it has found its ground in you and taken root.

Meanwhile, set boundaries.

Tell your friends you need time to integrate. If they need details, tell them what you've seen happen to others at the Casa without giving away your own experience. Keep your healing experience private.

Some ways to do this are to say that you've been on retreat, to a place where you've unplugged and unwound. Everyone understands this. You can say you're still integrating your experience and need lots of alone time. Ask for their support in your process. Let them know you'd like to connect after you feel more integrated.

Building community

Do you know people who've been to the Casa?

Did you make new friends or acquaintances while you were in Abadiania?

Share and process your experience with them. It's a great way to build community with those who understand the place and experience. When you give and receive support in this way, it keeps your healing alive and flowing.

I've changed! Now what?

Just as a caterpillar gives itself to its process of becoming a butterfly, you're metamorphosing into your self in a whole new way. Give yourself over to the process. Flow with it. Open to it. Let it take you to places you've never dreamed of going.

The more open you are, the further you will go. Notice your shifts and little or big miracles. You might feel like a new world is opening up for you. It is! It's a new you!

You might be more perceptive and intuitive. Tune in to what you're receiving. You may want to write things down to review later, especially if you have an active skeptic in you.

You might feel as though your identity and everything you knew is being completely overhauled. Rewired. Your life. Priorities. Relationships. Work. How you are in the world. Who you are.

Your soul may come forward. You might find something meaningful and sacred to be the center of your being and your life. You may reorient around something completely different.

Go with it. Let go of everything you don't need. Open to your new self and new experiences and the relationships entering your life. This is what transformation looks and feels like.

You are always connected to the Entities. They always work with you. Keep asking them for their support, healing, and guidance. They continue to help you unfold into your Beauty, Magnificence, Power, Joy, Grace, Love, and Light.

Open to the magic. To possibility. To Light and Love.

And offer up your gratitude to the wonderful, joyous beneficence and grace of the Entities—Beings of Light and Love.

Blessings to you, Dear One, on your journey.

GLOSSARY

Two o'clock line

A line in the afternoon session that you're invited to by the Entity.

Eight o'clock line

A line in the morning session that you're invited to by the Entity.

Entity

The Entity incorporating in Medium João's body. Although multiple Entities can incorporate during a Casa session, only one can use Medium João's body at any moment.

Entities

The phalange of Entities of Light and Love, directed by St. Ignacio, who work through and are channeled by John of God.

First time line
A line to go before the Entity if it's your first time at the Casa and you haven't had a distance healing.

Incorporation
The process of Medium João channeling an Entity.

Medium João
The man, João Teixeira de Faria.

Revision line
The line to go before the Entity seven days after your surgery/spiritual intervention.

Second time line
A line to go before the Entity when it is not your first time. If you've had a distance healing before visiting the Casa, you will need to go in the second time line since a distance healing counts as a pass before the Entity.

Spiritual intervention
See surgery.

Surgery line
The line for surgeries or spiritual interventions. You are prescribed surgery by the Entity or you may volunteer if you feel so guided, if and when your line is invited.

Surgery
A healing treatment where your spiritual aura is opened in order to heal, cleanse, and clear what you're ready to let go of and

release. It also brings forward your talents, gifts, and potential, and aligns you with your soul potential and purpose. There are two kinds of surgery: invisible, which ninety-nine percent of people have, and visible, for which you can volunteer.

RESOURCES

Books

John of God by Heather Cumming and Karen Leffler

The Book of Miracles: The Healing Work of João de Deus by Josie RavenWing

The Miracle Man by Robert Pellegrino-Estrich

Cosmic Healing: A Spiritual Journey with Aaron and John of God by Barbara Brodsky

A Little Book About Believing: The Transformative Healing Power of Faith, Love, and Surrender by Cash Peters

Gail Thackray's Spiritual Journeys: Visiting John of God by Gail Thackray

John of God: Journey to the Spirit World by Kelsie Kenefick

João de Deus by Jean Michel Robreau (in French)

Casa de Dom Inácio Terminology and Protocols

Official Casa Guide

Books on Spiritism

Allen Kardec
The Spirits' Book
The Medium's Book
The Gospel According to Spiritism
Obsession by Divaldo Pereira Franco (another famous Brazilian medium like John of God)
Family Constellations by Divaldo Pereira Franco

Spiritist books channeled by Chico Xavier

(Available on Amazon and in the Pencil of Light Bookstore, Abadiania)
Nosso Lar
The Messengers
And Life Goes On
Missionaries of the Light
In the Domain of Mediumship
Workers of the Life Eternal
Action and Reaction
In the Greater World

Spiritism and Psychotherapy

Kardec's Spiritism: A Home for Healing and Spiritual Evolution by Emma Bragdon
Resources for Extraordinary Healing: Schizophrenia, Bipolar and Other Serious Mental Illnesses by Emma Bragdon
Spiritism and Mental Health: Practices from Spiritist Centers and Spiritist Psychiatric Hospitals in Brazil by Emma Bragdon
Spiritual Alliances by Emma Bragdon

Past Life

Many Masters, Many Lives by Brian Weiss
Through Time into Healing by Brian Weiss
Miracles Happen by Brian Weiss
Messages from the Masters by Brian Weiss
Only Love is Real by Brian Weiss
Same Soul, Many Bodies by Brian Weiss
Mirrors of Time by Brian Weiss

Remarkable Healings by Shakuntala Modi
Memories of God and Creation by Shakuntala Modi
Testimony of Light: An Extraordinary Message of Life After Death
    by Helen Greaves
Memories of Afterlife by Michael Newton
Destiny of Souls by Michael Newton
Journey of Souls: Cases of the Afterlife by Michael Newton
Life between Lives by Michael Newton

Extraordinary Healings

Dying to Be Me by Anita Moorjani
Proof of Heaven: A Neurosurgeon's Journey into the Afterlife
    by Eben Alexander

DVDs

I do not Heal. God is the One who Heals: A Tribute to John of God Healing
John of God: Visiting João de Deus at the Casa de Dom Inácio
Nosso Lar
Chico Xavier Directed by Daniel Filho
The Mothers of Chico Xavier

Online resources

http://www.friendsofthecasa.info
http://www.abadianiaportal.com. A comprehensive website on
    everything about visiting Abadiania and the Casa
http://www.allan-kardec.org
http://www.spiritist.us/sss

Spiritist Centers in the San Francisco Bay Area

http://www.sfspiritistsociety.org
http://www.chicoxavierspiritistsociety.org/centers.html
http://www.nossolarspiritistsociety.org

ABOUT THE AUTHOR

MYTRAE MELIANA, MFT (pronounced "my-thray-yee") is a psychotherapist, hypnotherapist, soul midwife and speaker. She helps people heal, transform, and awaken to their soul's calling. Her own healing journey led her to John of God, and now she takes groups there. She is an award-winning writer and blogs about healing and transformation. She has a private practice in San Francisco. Visit the author online at www.mytrae.com.

If you enjoyed *John of God*, please consider taking a few moments to leave a review or rating at the retailer where you purchased it. Your comments help other readers discover great new reads and really do matter.